1

The Balanced Body
Move well – Train Better – Avoid Injury

First Edition

Jason Kelly B.S.
Exercise Physiologist

If you would like to contact me about seminars, workshops or further education, please contact me at:

tbblife.com

Visit this website for video and further support about the concepts in this book.

The Balanced Body
Move Well – Train Better – Avoid Injury

Foreword by: Dr. David Katz

Illustrations by: Jason Kelly
Cover Image by: Jason Kelly and Karla Patricia Barbosa Kelly
Interior Photos by: Karla Patricia Barbosa Kelly
Back of the book cover photos: Public domain photos by, pixelbay.com

Copyright © 2016 Jason Kelly
ISBN-13: 978-1530569915

First Edition
First Printing, March 2016

Printed in the United States of America

Acknowledgements

Writing a book takes time, dedication and perseverance to develop your thoughts and ideas. Therefore, I need to thank those who were patient in allowing me to achieve my goal. Writing a book was not only a personal achievement it was about sharing my teaching, knowledge and experience in health and movement for 19 years till present today. So, thank you to my wife Karla for believing in me and helping me with the photos in this book; clients over the years for their trust and business, allowing me to help them with their pain and issues; and to my mom and Jerry for all their confidence.

TABLE OF CONTENTS

FOREWORD

"True wisdom is on display when the detailed knowledge of a subject, and the myriad insights of long experience, are blended into a clear, compelling, and fundamentally simple message. *The Balanced Body* offers just such wisdom. Drawing on his training in exercise physiology and massage therapy, informed by years of hands-on clinical care, Jason Kelly artfully reveals simple, empowering truths about healing forces at our disposal, and the essence of healthful movement. This is an empowering book, offering millions an opportunity to eliminate pain, and cultivate vitality."

David L. Katz, MD, MPH, FACPM, FACP
Director, Yale University Prevention Research Center
Griffin Hospital
Medical Contributor, ABC News
Author, 'Disease Proof' -
Director, Integrative Medicine Center at Griffin Hospital
Editor-in-Chief, Childhood Obesity
President, American College of Lifestyle Medicine
President & Founder, Turn the Tide Foundation, Inc.

PREFACE

"My interest is in the future because I am going to spend the rest of my life there." – Charles F. Kettering

This book pertains to you if:

- you suffer from chronic back, joint and muscle pain, musculoskeletal disorders, immobility or inflexibility...
- you cannot breathe well or suffer from breathing disorders...
- you are a corporate office worker who sits at a desk all day long...
- you are a physical therapist, athletic trainer, chiropractor, strength trainer, performance coach, yoga or Pilates instructor or massage therapist...
- you are sick of being tired, suffering from fatigue, frustrated by feeling old and want to turn back the clock to regain youth...
- you are a part of the aging population and want to stop aches and pains…
- you are an athlete who wants to increase your performance and to reduce your risk of injury...
- or you just want to learn how to move better, be more efficient, healthier, fitter, and better prepared for fitness programs.

If so, then *The Balanced Body* is for you.

We are born and do not have any guide or manual on how to breathe or move. We depend on our culture and society to teach us but that has not been a successful approach. No clear defined way has ever been taught to us. Over the years' modern life, sitting too much and changes in our habits produced poor posture, misalignment, strain and pain, changing, compensating and evolving the way we breathe and move for the worst. All these ramifications' have led us to move less increasing the statistics of disease, disorder and affliction. And from the change in habits, we lost the natural functional programing that produces good health and movement. This is the reason why issues, like aches, pains, disease, disorders and conditions affect millions of Americans and people around the world today. Disease, musculoskeletal disorders, chronic pain, injuries, inflexibility, back and joint pain; have all evolved from the modern and sedentary lifestyle. As modern life and technology continue to improve and advance, the functional abilities and movement skills of the human body will devolve, evolving sedentary life. We need to be mindful of what we do each day to prepare for the next producing either a highly efficient or else a substandard, poorly functioning system through time. The missing piece in our evolution is being functional first. Looking at the statistics today, poor functioning is the chronic theme. But I am here to tell you that all this can be prevented and reversed.

Based on my work as an exercise physiologist and massage therapist, working with thousands of people over the past nineteen years, pain, injury and disorders are not the enemy. They are the results of faulty alignment and ineffective breathing that develop a path of poor quality, deficient and inhospitable to life. Thanks to these experiences and discoveries, I was able to help my clients lead a pain-free life, restoring their natural functional operating systems to move well. They overcame the same afflictions that affect the millions of people around the world. I realized that in order for them to appreciate and develop their health, strength, youth and vitality, they needed to move well. But they needed to be mindful of their inadequate habits that were unseen producing fatigue, pain, inefficiency and mediocrity daily. If not, the years of inefficient and ineffective programing would keep enabling their pain, injury, disease or disorder. By performing my manual therapy sessions on clients called 'Breathe, Stabilize, Move Function First', pain was eliminated instantly. And from the instant elimination of pain, range of motion, flexibility and mobility immediately returned and improved. When you restore alignment, you eliminate the issues and difficulties that constrain youth, energy and the ability to move well. This method proved to be so successful that I developed it into a self-care routine for all to learn and it is the inspiration in writing this book.

My clients over the years came from a wide variety of populations: from eliminating joint and muscular pain, people whom had past surgeries, injuries, people who have had musculoskeletal disorders, arthritis, the corporate office worker restoring their posture and alignment from sitting all day long to the apparently healthy population. I have worked with senior citizens, helping them to restore their youth, assisting them to move more and better. I have worked with professional athletes to improve movement, performance and range of motion, for example veteran baseball player Gary Maddox and the principals of the Pennsylvania Ballet. I also worked with world-renowned chef Georges Perrier and sports team owner Ed Snider. Whoever you are and whatever you do, you need to breathe, to stabilize, to move. It is how daily movement tasks, training and movement function, producing preventative and qualitative results to strength, fitness and health. I started to realize in writing this book that this knowledge is not just for those people who are suffering and have issues. This book is for everyone involved in fitness, exercise, movement and sport or for normal life. We all breathe and move unconsciously. It's automatic. However, if we are not breathing and functioning *well*, then we cannot move *well and frequently*. We need our ability to move for a very long time so we need to preserve its mechanics and functions. Breathing and alignment are the functional foundation and link.

From working successfully with all my clients over the years, I started leading workshops teaching Functional Movement Progressions for Movement and Sport. My first workshop with Villanova University athletic trainers and physical therapists was a great success. It led to other invitations addressing other local physical therapists and their staff. It was at this time I decided to create a simple guide that would be endorsed and used by experts in the field. This book, *The Balanced Body,* is targeted at the general public, athletic trainers, physical therapists, strength trainers, personal trainers, coaches, massage therapists, chiropractors and athletes. The exercises in this book are simple and the book is written for all to understand without technical jargon. The information and exercises in, *The Balanced Body,* will free your mind and body from the dependency on devices and misinformation. Traditional pain reduction approaches, like surgery and devices, or strength programs like yoga, are often counter-productive. Surgery and devices for example, stop pain, but create limitations in ranges of motion and compensations to movement. Strength training does not improve your misalignment and pain. It makes it worse! Your body is a machine. Like the many parts of a machine working together, they need to run smoothly and consistently without problems over time. When one part of the machine is not operating or functioning properly, strain occurs through the whole system and the results are ineffective and unproductive. Each day the machine is functional the more productive it will and can be. The more efficient your breathing and alignment, the more effective the body functions. The better the body functions, the more you can move with little risk to pain and injury. The more you can move, the more health, fitness, strength, youth, energy, vitality and vigor you can develop, leading to a greater longevity

The first secret in *The Balanced Body is* learning to harness the power of your mind, to become mindful. In order to breathe better, we need to be mindful of our breathing to change. In order to move better and stop pain, we need to be mindful of our alignment to transform. How many times have you thought about how you are breathing or your alignment today? We need to create habits that are progressive, not habits that strain and design decline. The mind needs to change the way it operates to affect the body, not just change the body. We don't need overcomplicated positions, exercises and programs to be healthy, strong and fit.

All of us, young and old, have the same lungs, joints and muscles. It is what we do through time that makes us healthy or not, preserves youth or speeds up the aging process, making us feel energetic or tired. We all have the same ability to achieve optimal health, strength and fitness. We all have the same capabilities to turn back the aging clock, preserve youth, and reverse disease and disorder. It is all about choices and what we do. You are never too young to maintain youth – and the sooner you start the better. You are never too old to regain youth. It is never too late to stop pain. The recommendations you will learn in *The Balanced Body* are your important first steps. The choice is yours.

"Life is really simple, but we insist on making it complicated." – **Confucius**

INTRODUCTION
"I move, therefore I am." – Haruki Murakami

From working with a diversity of populations, I made the discovery that everyone needs to be functional first. Pain and disorders, like musculoskeletal, are something we are not predisposed to; it is a faulty path we create from sitting, misalignment and from the modern and sedentary lifestyle. For example, as a child you breathed through the nose but as you became older, the modern and sedentary lifestyle switched breathing from the nose to the mouth, which is a very dysfunctional way to breathe. Breathing through your mouth makes you feel old, tired and you can't perform well or for long due to a lack of endurance. You probably equate your fatigue to something else other than breathing through your mouth, making you take pills, supplements and medications to have energy. After performing the breathing techniques in this book, you will feel great, awakened and can perform more and better. The same goes for restoring alignment, reversing pain and strain. By becoming aware and mindful to these functions you can control and transform them to have a direct impact on how you move, your energy, health and strength. You are only as healthy as you can breathe and as strong as your alignment can move. *"Natural forces within us are the true healers of disease."* – Hippocrates

The purpose of the Breathe, Stabilize, Move, Function First method, is to connect and integrate the respiratory, musculoskeletal and central nervous systems power. By synthesizing breathing, alignment and stability into exercises, you integrate all the systems to perform powerfully as one. The intention of the Breathe, Stabilize, Move, Function First method, is to create synergy producing a greater level of training, strength, health, fitness or sports performance safely and progressively. In contrast, weakness in one disintegrates the systems, leading to issues and imbalances affecting other systems, resulting in dysfunction. For example, breathing through your mouth decreases your volume of oxygen that leads to poor oxygen delivery to muscles, affecting the energy of the musculoskeletal system, making muscles tense, tired and inflexible.

The Breathe, Stabilize, Move, Function First method is setup in a step-by-step process restoring and developing your breathing and alignment to be functional, productive and effective. First, the book restores and develops your natural functional breathing process, nasal diaphragmatic breathing. Nasal diaphragmatic breathing strengthens your diaphragm to increase your volume of oxygen, lower your breaths per minute as well as lowering your heart rate and blood pressure because they are directly connected to how you breathe. It also makes you feel youthful, supports muscular contractions and flexibility, produces stability for the core and spine alignment, increases the power in the central nervous system and much more. You will also learn how carbon dioxide (CO_2) is needed in the body to utilize oxygen. Just one misconception taught by the media that CO_2 is toxic. It's not! After performing the breathing techniques you will learn that your mouth was meant to eat, not to primarily breathe. None of the aforementioned qualities can be achieved from mouth breathing.

Once you are breathing correctly, the corrective part of the book focuses on fusing breathing, stability and mobility into functional movement patterns to restore and strengthen alignment. The musculoskeletal system needs to produce stability to support alignment for the joints to function mechanically and optimally through range of motion. In variance, misalignment makes mobility limited, dysfunctional, inefficient and ineffective. But before you take on any corrective exercises, you will perform the Standing Postural Blueprint to assess your joints alignment. The pain and strain you experience is not primarily from the joint that has pain, it is from the joint that is misaligned in poor mechanical position that does not stabilize well weakening other joints. For example, the alignment of your hips determines the alignment of your spine and how your shoulders will function. Your pain may be in your shoulder but what's causing the issue is stemming from the hips.

After the corrective when breathing, stability and alignment are functionally integrated, you can progress range of motion though 5 levels. The exercises are simple. Instead of adding more exercises to your routine, here you add more mobility to your exercise on each level to move, train and progress. We need quality to produce quantity. Alignment is the quality and leverage that increases range of motion and power. You can move as far as you want through the levels or stay on the maintenance levels of 1, 2 and 3. It's up to you. There is even a routine for those who sit many hours a day called the Sitters Routine to stop pain and reverse sitting's detrimental effects. I recommend reading this book slowly and fully before you begin the method. This way you will understand what to do and be mindful before you do it. It is not about how fast and how much weight you can move, it is about how functional you are to move that produces' prevention and successful training progression. Slow movement allows you to screen for tension, possible injury potentials and train all the systems together into the movement to produce a pathway conducive for speed. On the contrary, speed adds more force to a joint in misalignment or to a muscle frozen and immobile that is detrimental to move.

The Balanced Body is not just another fitness, stretching, strength, power or mobility book. It is an evolutionary guide to make daily movement, fitness, stretching, strength, power and mobility programs functional, safer, more effective and progressive. There are too many programs today to improve health, fitness and strength, but not enough people to perform them safely and functionally. *The Balanced Body* is a unique approach to this age-old problem.

"The way you think, the way you behave, the way you eat, can influence your life by 30 to 50 years." – Deepak Chopra

Chapter 1
Why We Need Function
"Every human being is the author of his own health or disease."
– Buddha

Regrettably, as a society we have become more and more sedentary and dysfunctional in movement. Over the years, dysfunctional habits have silently corrupted our functional abilities to move. Lifestyles have changed and deactivated the body's natural functional power over the years from poor habits like sitting, misperceptions, carelessness, mindlessness and stress, and are evolving more rapidly. As technology develops and is imposed on society, its dependence will sit you into inactivity, getting more exercise from swiping your finger than from your body. Functional inefficiency leads to aches, pains, strains, injuries and disorders. In consequence, afflictions through time become worse and push us toward a more sedentary life. Whether you decide to move because you now have a disease, disorder or you are too sedentary, whether it is to be healthier or stronger, your body needs to be functional with breathing and alignment to be healthy and to move well. Society has been lead into illusion and misperception over the years.

The mind and body produce a functional integration, an operating system, of all the systems that interact and affect each other. This integration is non-physical and physical and interacts to create results. Like driving a car, the car drives (moves) based on how functions interact and produces a result; from physical components like having air in tires, the structural alignment of the frame, the axels, oil circulating through the motor and gas producing energy. The car will either drive well or poorly, similarly to how the body moves. If one part of the body is restricted in movement, if one system is not functioning properly, it affects all the functional systems losing interaction and integration with each other, affecting health and movement performance. For example, on the physical level, if the spine has poor posture (rounded spine), it restricts and limits it's own mobility and range of motion as well as the alignment and range of motion for the neck and shoulders. Joint positioning affects how other joints and muscles can and will move. A sub-functional inefficient system is formed that eventually leads to strain, pain, injury or disorders through time. On the unconscious level, the respiratory system affects the musculoskeletal and nervous systems. The musculoskeletal system affects the respiratory and nervous systems. The nervous system affects the respiratory and musculoskeletal systems. Change in one produces a change in all in an attempt to balance the deficiency or excess for good or for bad. The systems are regulated independently but their performance affects each other interdependently. For example, when you breathe through your mouth, you weaken and strain the respiratory system. A weak respiratory system strains the cardiovascular system by increasing blood pressure and the heart rate per minute making circulation and the heart work harder. It affects the musculoskeletal system by producing aches, pains, fatigue and tight muscles and destabilizes the nervous system making it feel stressed and panicky. It is finding and fixing the dysfunctional entry point that stabilizes and reconnects the cycle. If you drive your car with the parking break on the car strains to drive. Simply release the parking break and the car will drive functionally. When the body is free of limitations and restrictions, it will deliver a better functioning system, to perform and move daily leading to feel ageless and timeless.

In contrast, if the body is living in a dysfunctional state, it will progress into more disorder and dysfunction unless we change what is dysfunctional to be functional, what is not healthy to be healthy. Most of us place health and movement fairly low on the scale of awareness. People are not mindful of how they breathe, their alignment, posture or how they move. They just assume. People are **too** busy thinking about how to find shortcuts and the "path of least resistance" to achieve quick results, rather than appreciating the approach and importance of being functional. Being functional is more dependable, natural and leads to less stress and struggle to maintain health, fitness or performance rather than seeking the quick unnatural ways and shortcuts that are inefficient and temporary. They establish compensation and dysfunction in the body as well as dependency making what's natural seem like a struggle. If you seek out the functional ways to health, life and fitness, you will develop many systems together becoming stronger and powerful instead of unbalancing their functional state. It is the imbalance that causes the disintegration. What your body produces in function or dysfunction today holds the answers to your potential in your future.

Comprehend that movement is not bad for you. It is your present poor condition and habits; misalignment, muscle inflexibility, compensation and dysfunction that are bad for movement. Running, squats, presses, and push-ups are not bad for you. Your functional state is the missing piece of the puzzle. People simply do not function well, and as a result make themselves vulnerable to pain and injury. A dysfunctional system cannot support movement or strength training effectively nor progressively. But yet, you associate the faults of your pain and injury to movement, which is not the case. You can't drive a car if the axles are bent. You can't build a building on a foundation that is not level. Your body can't move well to develop health and strength if you have poor posture, joint misalignment, injury potentials and pain. Building strength and trying to maximize range of motion through these issues previously mentioned are how afflictions happen. The dysfunctional pieces do not fit into movement's functional puzzle. There is no functional sustainability for longevity; in contrast, this is what breathing, alignment and being functional bring to the table, prevention and movement longevity. The more functional and efficient something is the more effective it can be. It's about producing the quality first to sustain your quantity second. Evolving and enhancing your health and wellness becomes less complicated and more comprehended.

Movement is a necessity for prevention. For this reason, we need to attain function to preserve movement. Plato said, *"Lack of activity destroys the good condition of every human being, while movement and methodical physical exercise saves it and preserves it."* If health and life are not functional, then they will deteriorate over time, producing markers of aging, disease and disorder. The more you are not living well, the more you train your life to be that way. It disconnects the body's functional and mechanical abilities, disabling the use of the most effective and powerful weapon. That weapon is movement. We can erase and reverse these markers. The sooner erased the better. The longer the markers of aging, disease and disorder stay present it becomes habitual and disrupts health and life. Being functional, moving well and often activates and strengthens anti-aging mechanisms without disruption. It is what you condition yourself to be that writes the pages of your longevity.

INJURY STATISTICS

Health and fitness is a billion dollar industry. Pain and injury is a billion dollar business, with musculoskeletal disorders, joint immobility, poor posture, and back pain (especially lower back pain) as the chief complaints. Back pain is the leading cause of disability in Americans under the age of forty-five and affects more than 26 million Americans between twenty and forty-six years old (American Academy of Pain Medicine). But these issues not only affect the modern life Americans; they affect millions of people around the world like the plague.

Putting a Band-Aid over weakness, misalignment or pain only makes these issues worse. The problem today is that there is too much quantity. You can find lots of fitness, strength and power programs today. But there are not many people who have the functional integrity to perform them safely. There is not enough quality that goes into developing you first, preparing you for exercise, fitness and strength programing. People see, assume and try to mimic advanced movements, not understanding that breathing, alignment and joint stability are critical functions to perform strength programs and produce range of motion. As a former fitness director, I saw these common mistakes. The educational and functional approach that I provided showed clients and trainers you cannot assume what is faster and more advanced is better. This simply does not work with any misalignment or compensation on the smallest to the largest level. Two things can happen. You will either injure yourself or construct strength around your weakness that produces limitations in motion and affliction.

As a society, we do not practice prevention. Being mindful is how we prevent, evaluating how we breathe, checking our posture and alignment for the body. Prevention of pain and injury is really simple. It's about paying attention, understanding the present time, how and what to change in a positive, constructive and healthy way. When we are not aware or mindful, misconceptions will form and make us misconstrue our reality.

Misconceptions persist about strength, power, and quick weight loss—all issues that appeal to the ego to be unhealthy. Fitness and strength programs do not correct misalignments, back pain (especially lower back pain) or musculoskeletal disorders. Fitness and strength programming are meant to strengthen your current functional condition that you have attained. Those programs actually damage the compensated, misaligned body further. There are millions of people who do not have developed and evolved functional operational systems because of sitting too much, being sedentary or because of modern life. Comparing breathing through the mouth and misalignment to nasal diaphragmatic breathing and alignment is like comparing the Commodore 64 or first generation Windows to today's Apple OSX or Microsoft Windows 8. The Commodore 64 cannot run Skype or iTunes. It is our functional operating system (FOS) that instructs (runs) our movement programs, like strength, fitness, yoga and all others. If your FOS is not functioning properly, then there will be limitations in producing motion trying to do movements that you just cannot do naturally or properly.

We don't need muscle confusing programing, difficult positions and exercises to attain strength. These are just a few powerful misconceptions and illusions that lead to the high incidence of pain and injury. The problem is that movement, strength, fitness, sports, and power programs are being taught, shown on the Internet and sold to anyone who is willing to pay for them, but they are all offered without learning proper technique. Media and magazines perpetuate this type of thinking, failing to take into account how functional you need to be to perform those movements and programs safely and effectively. Society is just training the ego and not using the mind's rational approach. Society is declining and getting failing grades in function and movement. Society has scored A+ in Pain and Injury but an F in Function. We don't have programs that are effective at targeting the prevention of pain and injury. We only have programs to treat and rehabilitate them. Once you are injured, the system is altered, which is what we are trying to avoid. A body moving with misalignment is like trying to put a square peg through movement's circle hole. The pieces do not fit nor work well together; jamming, wearing and tearing each time you move from daily tasks to fitness and sport. Alignment is the prevention of pain, injury and wear and tear. I have witnessed far too many of these incorrect movements executed by fitness experts. These so-called experts are setting poor examples for society, just enticing your ego. We need the right role models to promote the ideal of function rather than selling a product just to create an image.

PAIN

Pain changes how you move and what you do. It changes your future movement plans and goals. It affects the entire nervous system. When pain is present, people compensate their posture, how they walk, run, stand, sit or move—anything to avoid it. They wait for it to just go away, not realizing what is actually happening. It causes other joints to adjust their position and muscles to compensate their function. Sometimes the pain will go away, but the issue is not solved. The fact is, you have unknowingly accepted the pain and unconsciously counteracted the position of the joints alignment.

The two different types of pain we will explore through this book are: the 'Why does my back hurt, I did not do anything to hurt it?' pain and pain that occurs through movement. They stem from the same root causes. The body's joints shift from alignment to misalignment for some reason, and that develops movement compensation.

In the first type of pain, the 'I did not do anything' pain, which is the most common, it is the development of poor habits or issues that get a little worse over time. A primary example would be from extensive sitting. You are only sitting in a chair but yet you are experiencing discomfort and pain. Discomfort and pain are felt because joint alignment becomes distorted and stability and balance become inadequate, producing a continuous and strenuous exertion on the body. Sitting for prolonged periods of time creates a loss of alignment, mobility and flexibility and diminishes range of motion. The ability to function as a whole is lost.

Misalignment is when joints lose stability and alignment; for example, poor posture, a rounded spine, tilted hips, a hyperextended lumbar or slouched shoulders, etc. The causes are due to strength imbalances, bad habits, poor ergonomics, pain, weak muscles or injuries. In misalignment, the joints adapt and maintain a position that is neither stable nor efficient through range of motion or movement. Joints cannot properly coordinate and synchronize movement because their functions have shifted from efficiency to inefficiency and balance to imbalance and it is unconscious to us until we feel aches or pains. Reciprocally, muscles and other joints will change the way they move. Muscles lose flexibility and develop isolated tension in the effort to support the joint misalignment, producing inefficiency at rest or through motion. Other joints and muscles shift to establish balance. Being unaware of compensation, joint misalignment and poor posture, loading movement programs, force or daily movement tasks on these issues, cannot support such intensity. This is how musculoskeletal disorders (MSD), pain and injury develop over time. It reaches a point where compensation starts to weaken, and you feel the aches and pains. Like the crumbling of a wall, over time, at a certain point, the wall loses the strength to sustain the tension caused by gravity and it falls to the ground much like the joints developing pain and injury.

The second type of pain is the same as the first, except you add forces to joint misalignment and instability through movement. This produces movement compensation with or without pain. For example, when squatting and the spine and shoulders round forward; when performing an overhead press and the spine has to bend to the side to lift the arm straight above your head or when lunging and the knee tracks inward or outward, etc. These are all signs that another joint is not aligned or stable, making another joint compensate it's position, deviating from it's aligned path. The lack of flexibility, an imbalance in strength, limited range of motion and instability are all results of misalignment. This unfortunately gets transferred into other movements and exercises because you don't feel anything is wrong. Anything out of balance or that does not have alignment imposes more force, meaning strain. As you move, you increase forces applied to the body. Moving fast or with speed increase those forces more. Alignment distributes these forces properly. Trying to perform a fitness or strength program on a body with poor function and misalignment, especially with speed, makes a good intention turn bad.

Movement compensation happens to protect you but it is not effective for movement in the long term. It is great that we have a system to adjust for weakness to avoid pain and injury. Joint compensation is the best tool the brain has to somehow create balance and efficiency. When one joint shifts they all shift to avoid pain, to provide reconfigured support. So, the misalignments start to feel correct because of the ensuing misalignment traveling through the body. Think of movement compensation like a spare tire, it is only for temporary use. Driving on the spare is only good for a certain amount of time before it wears down. You can only drive a few hundred miles before it gives out. It can only sustain a certain amount of force. The body has the same response. You can move joint compensations around successfully for some time but it does not mean it is effective for movement in the long term. It is definitely not effective for fitness and strength, loading force and intensity on joints that cannot stabilize and are out of balance. The problem is, you don't know you are compensating or in misalignment unless sensitivity, aches and pains are present.

On a different note, whenever pain is present, we move our body into asymmetrical and misaligned positions to make it stop because it is more comfortable. For example, with lower back pain, you see people standing, running and walking in awkward positions to minimize their pain. They counterbalance by producing poor posture, holding their body in a misaligned way to avoid the pain, adjusting from their natural aligned position. By reconfiguring joint alignment it will stop the pain producing an "inefficient balance". As time goes by, the body adapts to this inefficiency and it becomes faulty, defective and malfunctioning. When joints lose alignment they lose optimal mechanical position that produces structural strain. Misalignments become disorders that were not fixed or realigned.

Misalignments and movement compensations occur from;
- sitting all day, poor posture, shallow breathing, living the modern lifestyle,
- strengthening one side more than the other (asymmetry),
- moving, walking or running on a previous injury, pain or strain,
- isolated muscular strength training,
- repetitive movements.

Misalignments compensate joints to move in dysfunctional unnatural ways because misalignment can only move in limited ways.

According to Webmd.com, What Causes Musculoskeletal Pain?

The causes of musculoskeletal pain are varied. Muscle tissue can be damaged with the wear and tear of daily activities. Trauma to an area (jerking movements, auto accidents, falls, fractures, sprains, dislocations, and direct blows to the muscle) also can cause musculoskeletal pain. Other causes of pain include postural strain, repetitive movements, overuse, and prolonged immobilization. Changes in posture or poor body mechanics may bring about spinal alignment problems and muscle shortening, therefore causing other muscles to be misused and become painful.

How Is Musculoskeletal Pain Treated?

Different types of manual therapy, or mobilization, can be used to treat people with spinal alignment problems. For some acute musculoskeletal pain, these techniques have been shown to speed recovery.

According to Dr. Norman Marcus in the book *Back Pain Gone Forever,* "the primary source of 75 percent or more of back pain is from muscles not the spine". The issue manifests because your joints are misaligned and compensated functionally. Muscles are pulling tension in different directions from an unaligned joint, producing strength imbalances and asymmetry, creating a loss of equilibrium, likewise a loss of stability. Muscles feel strain and pain from the lack of balance and reciprocation, overloading them with tension. The seesaw effect of weight and tension imbalance, where one side is heavier than the other, makes a big difference to the body. The hips affect the spine. The spine affects shoulder mobility. What happens on the right side affects the left side and vice versa. Alignment creates function, optimal range of motion, energy transference for muscles to reciprocate, and for proper joint mobilization that results in effective strength. In misalignment, all this is inefficient, isolated and strained.

Each joint communicates to the next what it is doing and how it feels. The brain's cerebellum receives input from the joints, spine and muscles to maintain balance, timing and coordination for movement. It is an integrated feedback process called proprioception that you will learn more about in this book. Joints and muscles have sensors that affect alignment, how we stand, sit and move and sends the information to the brain. Proprioception produces the stability and mobility in each joint reflective of the position of other joints, efficiently or inefficiently. The second we lose alignment we fall into gravity's tractor beam pulling us further forward into imbalance. Gravity imposes a force. The brain and body need to learn how to balance and stabilize this force hence alignment is developed from this process.

As we experience misalignment we lose our natural functional way of moving well. These misalignments and dysfunctions produce detrimental effects and unhealthy conditions each day that lead to more serious conditions through time. Each day misalignment is present it becomes more powerful through time as a habit. As each day goes by the detrimental effects progress through phases of strain, pain, injury, disease and disorder, programing our future unless we change. Unfortunately, many of us hear the words safety and prevention and think it possess little value when it comes to strength training or physical performance. Yet, that is what strength training is suppose to do-boost safety and prevent pain and injury, augmenting the effectiveness of alignment to produce strength. You do not need to be a muscle-bound athlete to be strong. The problem society faces today, as well as any athlete is wanting big, strong lean muscles, but having poor underlying functional circuitry to attain and use them.

"When basic movement is limited or compromised, it follows the natural laws of energy conservation, compensation and avoidance of pain, avoidance of the unfamiliar, and the essential tendencies of survival." – Gray Cook, PT

Chapter 2
Misconception and Illusion
"We cannot teach people anything; we can only help them discover it within themselves." – Galileo

SITTING INTO DYSFUNCTION- THE NEW DISORDER

Sitting imposes detrimental effects on our body. But little has changed or been done to do anything about them over the years. Expensive chairs and devices make claims to help improve sitting posture but still fall short on their promises. It affects millions of people around the world: the corporate lifestyle sitting at a desk working on a computer, driving in a car, on a couch watching television for hours, flying on a plane, etc. It is spreading throughout our youthful generation today: playing gaming systems sitting hunched over for hours upon hours, being on the computer and telephone, addicted to social media sites and from sitting 6 to 8 hours in school. People of all ages are stricken by this disorder, ignoring and neglecting its detrimental impact and ramifications on their lives.

Sitting too much decreases energetic potential and capacity that creates fatigue. It slows down the metabolism of the body leading to feelings of laziness and tiredness. Taking a closer look at sitting from an inactive energetic standpoint, for every hour you sit you see a 46 percent increase in disability that affects your ADL, according to *The Journal of Physical Activity and Health*. ADL is your Activities of Daily Living that you perform as necessities for living each day (eating, walking, getting dressed, daily movement tasks around the house, at work and outside).

Sitting is the new disease and disorder because it is detrimental to your health, alignment and movement. We sit an average of 6 to 10 hours a day at a desk or on a couch. Sitting slows down metabolism that affects the body's ability to regulate internal functions. For example, sitting puts our health at risk for:
- *obesity and excess body fat.*
- *an increase in cholesterol, blood pressure and cardiovascular disease.*
- *an increase in blood sugar, exposure to hyperglycemia and type 2 diabetes.*

Sitting too much is now considered a risk factor for disease. A study done by Loughborough University and Leicester University with 800,000 people who sat for long periods of time throughout the day increased the risk of:
- *Cardiovascular (CV) event 147%*
- *Diabetes 112%*
- *Death from a CV Event 90%*
- *Death 4%*

Moving all day, performing more recreational activities, daily tasks and standing are now seen as better for health to maintain cellular and cardiovascular functioning. For this reason, standing and moving make the heart and muscles pump the blood more effectively than sitting. Because of gravity's pull, our body has muscle pumps to push blood throughout the body. When we sit, the blood stagnates and the muscles that pump the blood in the body are less effective and strain to do it. If we did not have muscles and the heart to pump blood, then gravity would pull and pool the blood. Blood is the lifeline that must circulate. If our body experiences too much antigravity from sitting then it strains the cardiovascular system making it difficult for blood to circulate, forcing the heart to beat more per minute and harder because of the ineffectiveness of muscles to help move the blood through the body. Gravity activates many functions in our body especially when it comes to the blood and the heart.

The body was not made or meant to sit or be sedentary. Sitting is a modern advancement that is good in some ways, but is the worst overall! When you sit, the respiratory, musculoskeletal and nervous systems become less active leading to inefficiency and dysfunction. Dysfunction through time leads to malfunction, that turns into a disorder or a disease:

- Sitting weakens muscles. This weakness destabilizes the body's joints impairing alignment producing pain and strain because of the lack of stability to maintain body alignment. Over time this leads to musculoskeletal disorders.
- Sitting compensates the center of gravity, the hips, that makes moving dysfunctional, which in turn, alters the energy and health of the nervous system because of the musculoskeletal strain produced.
- Sitting strains the respiratory and cardiovascular systems, increasing the heart rate and breaths per minute modifying how you breathe, causing the lungs to strain and breathe faster and shallower through the mouth disrupting oxygen levels.

When we sit too much, the body's systems and mechanisms become inefficient and less active, and its systems become stagnate where we experience fatigue and changes in organ, muscular and cellular functions because of the stagnation. Some systems are affected more than others. Each detrimental effect carries over to other systems, causing all to compensate. When systems deregulate and work harder, when muscles and joints destabilize, it causes others to pick up for their lack of function creating strain and imbalance, overworking producing fatigue. The antigravity effects produced from sitting, allows entropy to happen because of a lack of use and movement. The body needs to move. The lungs need to breathe. The blood needs to circulate. The muscles need to contract and stretch. The joints need to stabilize and move. All parts of the body need to move, as does information in the brain through the nervous system. When there is no movement, we see systems stop functioning well. We see this with blood sugar, cholesterol and obesity. Movement activates the systems functional mechanisms, just like turning on a light switch. That's why when you move, for example, blood sugar, cholesterol and obesity start to become normal again. If you don't change and move your body, the switch stays off and problems develop through time leading to deterioration.

The reason sitting has been categorized as a health issue is because of the work of Dr. Joan Vernikos. She was the former director of NASA's Life Sciences Division responsible for researching the health of astronauts and how space travel affected their body. It was great to find her research about antigravity and her comparisons in space and sitting's detrimental affects on our health. Her research is key because it shows that we can reverse and counteract aging and disease. The less we move, the more we sit, the less we use gravity and using gravity is essential. As she states, *"it is our lifeline"* and it activates our systems to function. She discovered that changes in bone density and muscle mass decreases about one percent per year on earth, where as losing one percent in space occurs in one week to one month, accelerating the aging process. Of course we don't live in space here on earth, but antigravity is highly associated to sitting and it's list of detrimental issues affecting our health.

Just because you workout one or two hours a day and you sit the rest of the day, it does not mean you are active, it actually is the opposite. Exercise only takes up a tiny portion of our day, about 30 minutes to two hours. That is simply not enough to balance the scales of sitting six to ten hours a day. It is more about perpetual motion, meaning; moving often performing daily tasks, like cleaning, cooking, standing watching TV, doing the Sitters Routine in this book, perform daily and recreational activities like taking the stairs, using longer ways to walk, walking instead of taking the car. Think of things that you can do that require standing and motion instead of using technology or something that requires you to be sedentary. For example, instead of ordering something on-line, go to the store and buy it. Try to remove the technology that has replaced the ability to move and explore. I feel curiosity has been lost over the years because modern life has made us more sedentary through technology, deactivating the body and using the brain less imprisoning the mind. We feel the need to have things instantly because of technology, making us less active. All this inactivity makes a difference mentally, physically, emotionally and energetically.

SITTING- STRAIN, PAIN AND DISORDER

Sitting is devolving the spine from it's upright position back into a hunched over position from using technology like cell phones and computers. It repositions and reconfigures joints, molding muscles to support their new misaligned position of a chair. It is a snowball effect that not only misaligns one joint it misaligns the whole body. This reconfiguration of joints limits and restricts mobility, flexibility and range of motion producing faulty movement. As you continue to sit hours upon hours a day you are training this position to stay and be dysfunctional, deactivating internal and external functions and mechanisms. The respiratory, musculoskeletal and nervous systems make adjustments and adaptations instantly over time to your energy, breathing and alignment not favorable to standing or moving.

First and foremost, from prolonged sitting the hip flexors, in the front of the hip, and a small muscle called Tensor Fascia Late (TFL), become tight. In contrast, the gluteus medius muscles, the muscles located on the sides of the hips, and the larger buttock muscles, the gluteus maximus muscles, the muscles on the backside of the hips, become weak. This is an excellent example of sitting's antigravity effects on the hip muscles. When we sit, antigravity takes affect on these muscles as well as the destabilization of the hip joints. This imbalance between tension and weakness (non-tension) causes the hips to tilt and destabilize, resulting in the loss of alignment. The hips are the center of gravity and foundation of support, therefore when the center of gravity is shifted, misaligned, or weakened, the whole body, the structural integrity and the joints compensate to produce balance located away from the center of gravity. This shift produces strain. For example, the lumbar spine's stability has to adjust and compensate to neutralize the misalignment from the hips, the hip tilt.

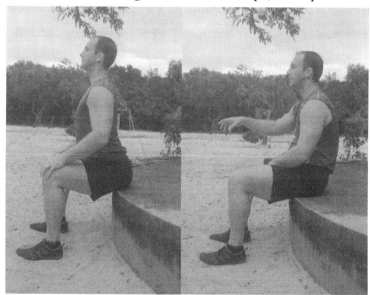 Depending on the position in which the hips (the foundation) shift or tilt depends on how the spine (the structure) compensates. The hip imbalance actually affects the whole spine because the hips and lower back are the foundational support for the spine. When the hips tilt forward (photo 1) the spine hyperextends. When the hips tilt back (photo 2), the spine will round forward. In turn, altering the alignment of the thoracic spine modifies the alignment and stability of the neck, shoulders and arms to a lesser degree of motion, limiting mobility. The thoracic spine is the platform on which the neck, shoulders and arms stabilize and move. You may think the pain in your neck and shoulders is the cause, but this not likely. The issue stems back to the hips. When you affect the hips and the lumbar, it furthers the path of dysfunction and compensation down through the legs, the knees and ankles as well. The process of misalignment and compensation transpires

throughout the whole body. We are unconscious to it because we only identify with things when there is pain. Restore alignment, stabilize it and range of motion and mobility will return as well as flexibility.

All the gluteal muscles' primary function is to produce alignment, stability and balance for the hips and lower back. Alignment sets off the stability and mobility chains in movement. Muscles contract to stabilize joints for other muscles to have a platform to stretch and for other joints to mobilize in movement. This process does not occur so well when you have misalignment producing poor stability and limitations in motion. It produces a ripple effect through the whole body. The longer something stays present, the more habitual it becomes. Habitual misalignments strain the respiratory, musculoskeletal and central nervous systems causing the body to work harder at rest. Your body adapts to live with this system.

When sitting for long periods of time throughout the day, the spine is the part most affected by excessive and extensive immobility. It is the first sign you see and feel, which is why you see the spine and back as the cause, not the hips. But it is the hips that are responsible for making the spine adjust from it's aligned position. Like I said before, it is not the joint in pain that is the problem, it is another joint in misalignment causing the issue. The classic pattern of misalignment for sitting is; a posterior hip tilt (hips tiled back) and a rounded forward spine like you just saw in photo 2 on the other page. The spine has a neurological connection to all the joints. Depending on what position the hips and spine are in will depend on how muscles and joints will be affected, impacting standing and moving.

As with a falling wall, we can buttress the wall in many different places to prevent the wall from collapsing, much like we do with our spine stabilizing poor posture. One minute you are slouching, the next minute you are sitting back, the next minute sitting with one shoulder higher than the other. As you try to move to eliminate discomfort, pain or tension in your chair, other joints are forced to move into compensation, compromising their integrity. The pain may stop but your alignment, posture and movement has become dysfunctional. You sacrifice posture and alignment to handle pain. Deficient posture and poor spinal position make the joints adjust their positions to support the spine. This changes the muscles' roles making their primary focus on staying tense, buttressing the spine to maintain a position of misalignment that switches flexibility and mobility to immobility. Furthermore, poor posture puts more pressure and force on the lungs because of the spine rounding forward. As the lungs feel more pressure, it causes you to breathe though your mouth making the lungs work harder than needed at rest. When the posture is poor, there is a reflex built in that compensates breathing to the mouth, and vise versa. When you breathe through your mouth, you breathe into the top of the lungs, where as nasal diaphragmatic breathing activates and uses the diaphragm and the abdominals to intake more oxygen into the bottom of the lungs. The bottom of the lungs, are larger than the top, where there is about 30 to 50% more capacity. Nasal diaphragmatic breathing has many benefits that not only pertain to increasing the amount of oxygen in the body, but that transfer physically for alignment and stability. Breathing is highly influenced from a life of sitting too much.

Most people sitting for long periods of time have poor posture that exacerbates back pain and sensitivity throughout their body. When this happens, this does not mean to go and do back bends or yoga cobras in an attempt to restore alignment and integrate the functions. That's how injury and strain happens, trying to move into range of motion when joints are restricted and limited by misalignment, and the functional circuitry is not so effective. As you restore the functional foundation to the hips and lower back, you will be able to perform those exercises and notice other aches and pains in the body subside and resolve as you unjam misalignment. The spine is an antenna where all the nerves innervate the brain and the rest of the body. If the spine is not functioning well and under stress and strain, the rest of the body will feel it. Sitting too much is a very important reason why people develop issues with their spine and body as they age. This is the importance of preserving the spine's alignment for energy, youth and vitality. Breathing, the spine and the joints are all interconnected. Breathing and alignment create an energy system linking the respiratory, musculoskeletal and nervous systems together. As for sitting, it weakens and disconnects their link.

The best way to balance sitting too much and modern life activities are by splitting them up throughout your day. You don't always have to sit and you don't always have to do things the easy way. This is what has been imposed on society and what we need a change from; modern life and technology making us lazy and tired, imposing dysfunction and imprisoning movement. The body adapts to what we produce and that creates a system. But we can easily transform this system to be more productive through a change of habits. If you can change habits from sitting too much, you can transform the biomarkers that create fatigue, aging, pain, disease and disorder. First, I need you to understand how to breathe, activate and strengthen the diaphragm, and establish joint alignment and stability to upgrade and restore a functional system.

TIPS FOR SITTING BETTER

- Avoid crossing your legs. It rotates one hip, constricting those muscles reprograming the neuromuscular system through the musculoskeletal, while the other hip is normal. This will affect your knee and shorten your leg.

- Stand more often when watching TV or at work. Make it a point to get up every 15 to 20 minutes (3 to 4 times and hour). The most important thing is to get up as frequently as you can. You can alternate sitting and standing throughout your day to create balance or perform a small routine that requires movement. When you stand up, take a few minutes to do two to three exercises to counteract sittings detrimental effects.

- Try to change your workstation to standing if you have the capability.

- Use a chair that allows you to lean forward and move your legs. I like to use a stool or backless chair for the freedom to sit in different positions, not depending on sitting back into a chair. Therefore I need to stabilize my body to sit.

- Sit on a firm surface for your pelvis. Roll the hips forward on your sit bones in the groin area. You will feel the gluteus medius contract and make the connection to the lower back. This will move your hips into a better, aligned position as well as improve the spine's posture and alignment. You can see this from the previous photos 1 and 2. You can keep your feet flat on the floor or straighten your legs stretching your hamstrings contracting your quads. It helps to solve a small piece of the problem. When you sit back into the chair, it rolls the hips back and the spine slouches.

- Sit up not slouched in the chair. Use a post-it note on your computer so that when you see the note it will automatically remind you and condition a positive habit.

- Use a towel when sitting in a chair that has a back at a desk. I have shown many corporate office workers how to do this. Take a beach towel roll it up. Place it between the middle of your back and the chair long ways, parallel, and lean back. It will keep your spine aligned and strengthen the muscles as your lean back. Lumbar devices don't work because its' not the lumbar that is the problem, it is the hips and spine creating the issue for the lumbar.

FLEXIBILITY- EVERYONE IS FLEXIBLE

People just stretch not realizing how and why muscles are tight. Stretching is just one part of the equation that is the least significant to flexibility. Flexibility has rules, not just stretching a muscle. Stretching a muscle without applying the other rules can produce pain, strain or little to no progression.

Flexibility is just one part of many ingredients for movement that makes it functional. When people hear the word flexibility, they think about stretching a muscle. This is correct, but it is not the sole basis of how flexibility functions. The flexibility of a muscle is based on the body's joint alignment. If a joint is misaligned, like a seesaw without equilibrium, then more tension is developed in muscles on one side more than the other, producing imbalance. Dr. Stuart McGill, an internationally recognized low back specialist, states it perfectly. Imagine a thin communications tower. It needs to be held straight up in the air by the tension of the guy wires. If those wires do not have equal tension, it will pull more in one direction, disrupting the balance and alignment of the tower and it will no longer stand straight. Now imagine tight hip flexors and weak glutes; tight chest muscles, a rounded spine and weak back muscles; tight hamstrings and weak quadriceps. In these examples, the joints have lost their alignment and center because muscles are pulling more from one side than the other, tugging the joints away from the center, tilting the scales to imbalance losing stability. Muscles lose flexibility, develop tension and decrease range of motion for a reason. (Specifically due to sitting, repetitive movements and isolated strength training.)

Without alignment and joint stability, muscles will maintain tension to preserve the stability and alignment that was lost by the joint, decreasing the muscle's ability to be flexible. It inhibits your potential to perform functional range of motion, making it difficult to perform a movement pattern, like a lunge, that requires alignment, stability and flexibility. Stretching a muscle that is "maintaining misalignment" or without understanding why means you are stretching inefficiency. This will not have progressive results or benefits. A change in habits and routines are required.

People say they are not flexible because they don't know how to be flexible. Their mechanics cannot function effectively because they are using an inefficient, compensated and subpar system for movement. Habits will alter function, like you previously read about sitting. It is a myth to say, "I am not flexible." In fact, everyone is flexible. I have proven this many times to my clients, producing instant flexibility in their body in just minutes. In reality, it is your proprioception system, the functional operating system that is not producing the alignment and reciprocation signals needed to move well and gain flexibility. Being flexible and moving well is not difficult and only requires some adjustment and change in your body. It's like computers. Old computers cannot run advanced programs effectively. Much like the misaligned, compensated body can't run flexibility programing effectively. Upgrading and enabling the system to function through alignment produces the quality to activate its attributes.

Try this movement to understand the principal of muscle reciprocation, contraction and stretch, for flexibility and how it works instantly. You can use this technique throughout the body and you will apply it in the movement section of this book. First, try to touch your toes and see how far you can stretch. Don't force. Just naturally roll down with your legs straight and do a classic toe touch. When the motion stops that's the marker. Feel for tension through the movement as well. Now, lean your hands against a wall or tree for support. Lift the toes off the floor contracting the muscles in the front on top of the ankles and the quadriceps. Keep the contraction of the ankles active by pulling the toes up toward the knees. Lean forward with your toes up, lift your hips up and slowly slide your hands down the wall or tree, moving toward the floor contracting the quads and stretching the hamstrings. When the stretch stops, hold the contractions and stretch together for 5 seconds and slowly come back up. If you cannot make it all the way down just hold the position breathe and contract the muscles.

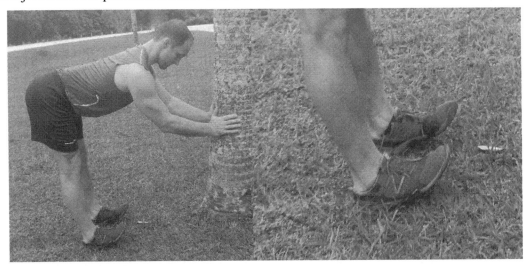

Now, do the exact opposite. Contract the quadriceps and do a calf raise picking your heels up off the floor. Shift the weight into the big toes. Bend forward slowly lifting the hips up to the ceiling stretching the hamstrings and contracting the calves and quadriceps

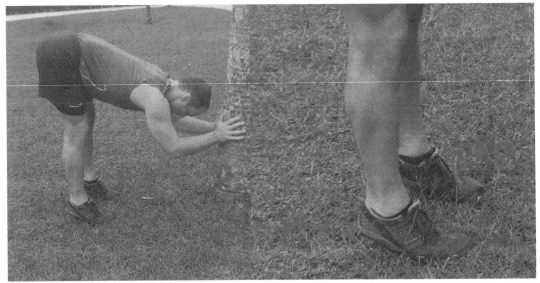

all together. When the stretch stops, hold the contractions and stretch for 5 seconds. Put your heels on the ground and slowly roll back up. Now, touch your toes again rolling down to the floor to feel and see your progress. It should be easier and you should have more range of motion to bend forward instantly. All you did was use contraction and stretch to balance muscle tension that produced a better, aligned position for the joints. Flexibility is not just about stretching. Contraction is an essential component because it guides and stabilizes joints into position for muscles to stretch. Try it for a few more repetitions to get the full effect. You can also use a slant board under your feet but I prefer to use your functional operating system to coordinate movement.

I have personally attained flexibility, not by only stretching muscles, but by contracting muscles to maintain joint alignment through a pose or movement pattern, for instance, contracting the quadriceps to stretch the hamstrings or contracting the glutes, the buttock, to stretch the hip flexors. The contraction of muscles guides and pulls the joint into alignment that allows range of motion to happen as well as increase, triggering the flexibility signal. This is why clients attain instant flexibility and move well. You enable the system to produce alignment and the functional mechanical advantage by contracting muscles to stabilize a joint, resulting in flexibility. It is similar to leverage. Training this process teaches you not to force flexibility or stretch on muscles that does a little bit of damage each time. It teaches you that flexibility and movement require alignment, stability and muscular contraction to stretch effectively to pass through range of motion. Like I said before, stretching a muscle is just one small component of producing flexibility. Alignment from a joint is a necessity to attain functional, resilient and optimal flexibility that also prevents over-stretching a muscle. Range of motion and flexibility is about working within your means and not trying to contort your body to move outside your ability. If you can only move 60 degrees from the horizontal with the shoulder joint, lifting your arm straight into the air above your head, you are missing out on 30 degrees of motion. You will have to compensate your alignment to move your arm into a 90-degree angle above your head. That's not correct, and applying a strength conditioning fitness program to the issue is definitely not the answer.

At 43 years of age, I have excellent range of motion and flexibility. Using joint stability (contracting muscle) will preserve alignment for muscles to stretch optimally and functionally, producing the correct process for flexibility, range of motion and movement progression. It produces resiliency rather than stretching or over-stretching a muscle. You want flexibility to be resilient and strong, not loose and flimsy. According to the Merriam-Webster Dictionary, resiliency is the ability of something to become strong again after something bad happens or the ability to return to its original shape after being pulled, stretched, pressed, bent, etc. Contracting muscles produces reciprocal tension that transfers to stretching muscles, creating a stronger, more resilient stretch. When it comes to flexibility this does not mean, go do yoga. Yoga is a form of movement that uses flexibility in its movement patterns. Many people get injured from performing yoga, not understanding their body, thinking to just stretch muscles. Yoga programing is all about breathing, stabilizing, contracting and stretching muscles to move

NEW APPROACH TO EXERCISE, FITNESS AND STRENGTH

There are some really great training programs available today. But before undertaking any strength program, it is vital that you take the right approach. In order to perform the best and most effective program, you must comprehend breathing, alignment and stability, your functional attributes, to interact with that program. As you increase your level of training, these functional attributes become a necessity. It is impossible to apply any weight training, strength, speed or power program to a body that does not function well, that does not have the structural foundation, circuitry and integrity. When you apply forces to physical and mechanical structures, like a building or a skeletal system of the body, you need to make sure that it can withstand those forces. The new approach to exercise, fitness and strength is not about speed or power it's about breathing, alignment, stability and function. Alignment provides the ability to withstand forces applied from strength training, running, daily movement tasks, fitness programing and sport performance. Alignment leads to good mechanics that function well, and functioning well leads to develop a healthy musculoskeletal and nervous system to produce quality movement as well as to maintain energy and stamina.

Society is so crazed with fitness, strength and health. People are so concerned about how they look and attaining strength that they sacrifice their health, vitality and functionality. Exercise, strength, and movement fads will always keep emerging. It is like a revolving door. Effective movement is not possible without alignment, and that rule does not change. If you have alignment, and know how to breathe, stabilize and move then you can participate in any strength program. Many strength training program's today are a reflection of society's lack of awareness with respect to functionality. The way to develop strength and movement is to understand yourself, your capabilities, weakness and limitations and fix those weaknesses and limitations. They are the issues that develop pain and injury and block development and progression. Yet this level of understanding is something programs most often do not offer. The weakness and limitation in your mechanics and function will only present a problem as you load weight, force, speed and strength to the dysfunction. When you build strength on a body that has a weak structural foundation or if there is an unconscious weak point, it will not withstand the strength augmentation through time. As forces increase and strength goes up, the weakness (misalignment, asymmetry, poor posture) becomes weaker that cannot withstand more force or tension.

There are many cookie-cutter programs out there, but bear in mind, what may best work for you, is based on your weakness. If you are not functionally efficient, a cookie-cutter program will create very little progress and harm for you. One program cannot be applied the same to everyone. If you have poor posture and the program wants you to perform presses, pull-ups, pushups and squats; your shoulders, spine and knees will take a lot of abuse from loading mechanical disadvantages with that poor posture. This is something strength training and boot camp-type programs like to perform in their programing on you. Try this simple example to gain insight into the thought here. Slouch your shoulders and round your spine. Create temporary bad posture, if not so already (photo 1). Slowly, without force, lift your arm up as high as it will go above your head (photo 2). Bring the arm down. Now, sit up or stand up straight lifting up your chest (photo 3). Lift your arm up as high as it will go, again without force (photo 4).

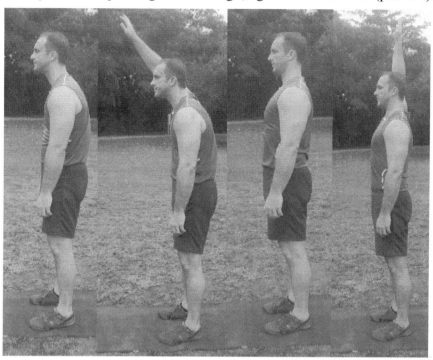

You may not have been aware how this works. Where there is misalignment there is unconscious adaptation. The point I wanted you to see is the power of activating awareness to make the unconscious conscious, developing mindfulness of your alignment as you move, as you will experience through this book. If the spine has poor posture the shoulders' lose the ability to function and produce range of motion. You can't simply lift your arm straight above your head, but yet, you probably don't feel pain when lifting the arm because you compensate to do it. If your hips are tilted forward when you run, jump, etc., the lower back absorbs a lot of force. I want you to be aware of your body before you participate in these popular programs like yoga, boot camps, high intensity training and maybe CrossFit. Not being mindful of your poor posture, shallow breathing, your shoulder joints' mobility or that of all the joints of the body to function, limits them and puts them at risk to injury. Anyone can produce strength. But in a misaligned body, strength makes a misaligned joint stronger, but stronger with imbalance, instability, limited mobility and decreased range of motion. If the joints don't have alignment, joint misalignment is going to be your weakness.

You can see how just one simple compensation, such as the spine's posture, affects alignment and the quality of movement. It is the compensation that is going to have a limiting effect on your movement development. You will move as best your alignment knows how, limited or functional. As you can see, when you train with joint misalignments and imbalanced strength, your strength training will work against you. This is why it is so important to be functional and efficient and why we need a new strength approach. You don't need to become another number in the rise of sedentary and injury statistics. Contributing to the rise of injury statistics is the misinformation disseminated by magazines, TV and the internet, that fail to educate people about how to correctly prepare the mind and body in strength training.

The new approach to strength is using the Breathe, Stabilize, Move, Function First Method to develop a power source, a functional operating system, to be efficient first. Alignment unlocks range of motion, flexibility and mobility. Misalignment locks and limits range of motion, flexibility and mobility. When you **sit** in a strength machine, like a chest press, leg curl or bicep curl, etc., you lose the stability of joints and only contract individual muscles that end up producing an imbalance in strength. There is no synergistic interaction with other muscles and joints working to produce the linkage through the body that strength requires. This type of training imbalances the musculoskeletal and neuromuscular systems, as well as not using the respiratory system optimally to produce pressure in the core for stability to move. The body has to learn how to stabilize to move without a machine, using its alignment and balance to improve coordination.

As you can see movement is third in the sequence: breathe, stabilize, (core/alignment), then move. Most people practice only strength training and movement, ignoring the first two necessary components, i.e., breathing and (alignment) stabilizing. Quantity is easy. Anyone can run fast down the street. Anyone can hoist a weight. But can you do it well with quality that works to create quantity safely, repetitively and consistently? Increasing strength is about production over time. Whereas in many strength and power programs, over time, strength production goes down but you continue to perform with poor technique, shallow breathing and misalignment, deactivating your functional system. Understand that when form is gone, you are overtraining from a point that does not yield results. When breathing and posture are lost, that is the sign that the central nervous system is tired and needs time to rest and recover.

Trying to do new exercises or progress movement without having mastered basic techniques first will falter because you don't have the ability nor the skills to progress movement without the functional circuitry. You cannot apply strength conditioning programs under the assumption that people are functional, especially in a society that is dysfunctional. Why take the risk? It's time to practice synergistic methods and to include timing, coordination and synchronicity of breathing, core stability, joint stability joint mobility and proprioception to yield strength results. I am not trying to sell you on a quick fix method. I am trying to sell you on your own natural functional ability for progression that delivers quick results.

Chapter 3
Functional Efficiency: The Art of Function
"Knowing is not enough; we must apply. Willing is not enough; we must do." – Bruce Lee, quoting Goethe

THE PROPRIOCEPTION SYSTEM: BRAIN, THE HUMAN GPS

Proprioception is power. We all can tap into this power locked in the unconscious mind. Strength, power and movement are ninety percent mental. Why? Strength, power and movement are all powered by the unconscious functions of breathing, stability and alignment. The proprioception system is an intuitive, unconscious system that we can tap into through awareness and mindfulness, to make it conscious.

The proprioception system is comprised of nerve receptors located in muscles, joints, tendons, ligaments and skin throughout the body. Its job is to perceive fluctuations in strength, posture, breathing, alignment, flexibility, tension and pain. The proprioception system owes its intelligence to a feedback loop, where data comes to the brain about the muscles and joints, allowing it to arrange a pattern for them to stand or move based on this information. When it senses tension in a muscle or a joint in misalignment, for example, it sends a signal back to the brain to adjust for the compensation without feeling any pain. One of the proprioception system's jobs is to monitor TPIPS (Tension, Pain, Injury Potentials). It can be positive or negative feedback and adaptations happen in an instant. It is of the utmost importance to clear tension and pain, and create alignment and balance for proprioception to maintain the system each day. The longer immobility, sedentary life, misalignment and pain fester, the more they create compensation, the further it influences the development of habits and a subpar dysfunctional system. The good thing about compensation is it protects you from harm, pain and injury. The bad thing is, it does it unconsciously and is not effective for movements made in daily life and fitness performance. Once injury happens the system is altered, made weaker, which is what we are trying to prevent. Until we become conscious of the proprioception system, it will act dualistically, like anything that is unconscious. The movements we do, the postures we create, the mouth breathing we use, the cause and effect, have results. We can control and predict these results and outcomes. Mindfulness provides this control.

For example, I have worked with many corporate people who sat all day long at a computer. All of them were not mindful to how they were breathing, their posture and how they were sitting. They just understood the tension, strain and pain they were experiencing each day. I was able to restore their natural breathing through the nose and rebalance and realign their body in one or two sessions and thus rid them of strain, back pain and tension. It works that fast. By the next time they came back, they were imbalanced again because the brain and proprioception system adjusted to maintain their habitual sitting position. The brain adopted a program based on a habitually seated, sedentary lifestyle over the years. This is a big part of the problem. You learn to move and function daily from the seated position, using this as a functional operating system. I simply prescribed these individuals with a 10-minute program to perform often at work during the day without losing time or productivity. Basically things you can do at your desk. The program is meant to simply remove the "stick from the spinning wheel" to maintain alignment for the hips and spine instead of falling into joint compensation. Those who practiced were successful at stopping pain and moving better. Unless reversed, compensation and dysfunction will imprison your ability to move well. Remember, if you train inefficiency you become inefficient. If you train and move with poor posture and misalignment, you are training and moving limitations. Awakening to the situation is a must.

How can the office worker sit day after day with misalignment and poor posture or run, strength train and move efficiently and effectively? The answer is: he can't. He can't keep loading misalignments, compensations and dysfunctions unconsciously daily. A joint under misalignment is under the influence of gravity that increases the pounds of pressure on a joint. When you move, the forces applied increase the pounds of pressure even more on misalignment. The joints are being exposed to an increase pull of gravitational force from poor alignment. Misalignment produces instability and imbalance with weakness on one side and strength on the other that produces strain. Alignment transfers and distributes forces properly using stability.

Signs of dysfunction in proprioception and not being mindful of movement:
- Awkward walking gait.
- Sitting too long throughout the day.
- Have poor posture, a rounded spine.
- Overtraining.
- Trying to force stretch or contraction.
- Using 100 percent of force all the time with small and heavy weights instead of learning how to control the force.
- Letting the force control you.
- Not being able to contract certain muscles on command.
- Isolated muscle training.
- Being unskilled in conserving energy in movement training.
- Being unable to leverage the body with muscles and joints.
- Lacking coordination and balance.
- Breathing through the mouth, shallow and rapidly.

We evolved the brain, so now it's time to re-educate and re-write its functional software. Learning to breathe, strengthen alignment, stabilize and perform movements slowly; will create mindfulness and connect us to proprioception for functional efficiency. Once you develop a functional system, you can add intensities and speed because the system knows how to function to sustain them. Use slow movements to make your brain fire signals consciously for muscles to contract and stabilize joints, for muscles to be flexible and other joints to move. By actively contracting muscles, the proprioception system can be conscious and informed to restore alignment and provide flexibility as well as release tension in other muscles. This should be habitual training. Performing movements slowly produces the circuitry to do it fast and prevents affliction. Performing movements slowly will consciously show any inconsistencies that affect mobility and movement. But if you do movements fast without the functional circuitry, then you are at risk.

It's rare to think about things that are involuntary. We are rarely conscious of breathing through the mouth and misalignment. When something compensates from the norm it does not mean it will automatically reset. It means the brain is going to adjust, adapt and change until you find the issue. Everything will start to form around this process. You have to be mindful, intervene, practice and change. I want you to feel it to believe it, which has more power than just reading the words on a page. What's more important is to help you understand the unconscious mind and make it conscious. The power in the unconscious mind goes beyond things we can consciously see, to make real what we can only imagine.

Breathing, stability and alignment are the keys to entering the proprioception system, making the unconscious conscious and functional.

WHAT IS FUNCTIONAL EFFICIENCY (FE)?

How you move, how you live and how you eat all tell a story about your wellness. We practice this primarily through physical activity and nutrition. We know how to do it, but why are people not doing it, living a functional healthy life?

Frequently, it is reinforced that faster is better, that you don't need to spend time with technique and practice to achieve a goal in health or fitness. This in particular, is what magazines' and the media portray. Their methods, plans and advice are more attractive and dysfunctional than practical and beneficial. They teach us how to be dysfunctional and unhealthy for overnight success, suppressing sustainability to prove a point using the quantity over quality principal. In consequence, mindfulness and consciousness have been disconnected and compensated, sacrificing our functional abilities to move, have energy and be well. All in all, this destines you to dysfunction, disease and disorder, making you dependent on unnatural ways.

Function is a natural purpose to train, work or perform to be useful. For example, breathing functionally strengthens the diaphragm to increase the volume of oxygen and to establish stability between the abdominals and spine. Joints function for stability and mobility. Muscles function by stretching and contracting.

Efficiency is the achievement of maximum productivity without wasting energy. Efficiency is when your body can perform certain tasks, from digestion to movement, without expending a lot of energy or wasting energy. For example, alignment, balance and coordination produce efficiency during movement; exercise lowers the heart rate and blood pressure, etc.

Functional Efficiency is the integration of breathing, joint alignment, stability, muscular contraction and muscular flexibility, maximizing productivity and energy for movement without pain, strain or injury interfering.

Functional Efficiency – FE – is the integration of:
- Nasal diaphragmatic breathing activating and using the diaphragm.
- Joint alignment and posture.
- Muscular contraction to create flexibility and joint stability to preserve alignment.
- Muscular flexibility to stretch and produce range of motion.

For example, when you run or move faster than you can breathe or if you are gasping for breath in a high intensity strength and conditioning program, breathing through your mouth, this weakens and compensates FE. When you don't breathe properly, you are not using the diaphragm to produce the pressure needed for the abdominals to create stability for the spine, and you lose the ability to develop and increase volume of oxygen. Affecting the spine's stability and postural alignment ramifies its effects specifically to the neck and shoulders as well as to the other joints of the body disrupting their stability and mobility throughout the whole body and how it will move. Many issues for the spine, neck and shoulders, can be routed back to poor breathing dynamics and instability.

Another example is, when you breathe through your mouth, you do not use the inhalation (postural) muscles effectively. Breathing through the nose contracts the diaphragm that pulls down on the ribcage, causing those muscles to contract, as well as to produce pressure in the abdomen resulting in tension of the abdominal muscles to stabilize and support the spine. Breathing through the mouth weakens the inhalation muscles because you don't activate the diaphragm effectively breathing through the mouth, losing postural strength for the spine, neck and shoulders. Every breath you take affects the strength of spinal alignment. The strength of spinal alignment affects the entire joint system. You can decrease neck and back pain as well as shoulder pain by simply inhaling properly through the nose to breathe. Nasal diaphragmatic breathing and alignment are like catalyst reactions in chemistry. They set off a chain reaction in the body needed to unlock other functions for efficiency and effectiveness. Where as mouth breathing and hip misalignment servers the connection, limiting movement, producing energy strain and inefficiency, making the lungs work harder breathing into the space at the top of the lungs.

A third example is, when muscles develop strength imbalances. The weak contraction or the inflexibility of a muscle loses the ability to perform a full range of motion; like trying to extend your leg to contract the quadriceps and the hamstrings are tight. Or, if the muscles pull on one side of the joint more than the other, the muscles will pull the joint into misalignment when the strength or tension is more on one side; similar to the chest muscles being stronger than the back muscles, pulling the shoulders forward. It repositions the joint alignment affecting range of motion adjusting your proprioception. You see this a lot in high school athletes. They want to develop their chest and biceps that leads to pulling their shoulders forward out of the whole body alignment.

When joints don't work together, isolation creates a loss of function. Losing function is losing quality, and that is what teaches you how to move. This is why technique is important;

- to develop and run the functional software in your body;
- to prepare and develop the potential and ability for optimal movement; and
- to produce the proper mechanics and skills for maximizing strength or fitness training.

Taking on the functional approach will produce mindfulness and consciousness for your potential. Though it is possible to do anything you want and move any way you choose, you must first know the rules and the equations that create movement:

Breathing + Alignment + Stability + Muscular Contraction + Flexibility = Movement.

Movement is expressed as an equation because it has many functions that are integrated and interdependent to create one movement, like a lunge, squat, pushup, etc., even running. All these factors integrate in a coordinated, synchronous fashion to create natural movement. Consider these factors in training movement, techniques and patterns so that a balanced system can begin to function, emerge and work naturally for energy efficiency daily. If you don't use it, you lose it. When you lose it, you pick up unconscious, sloppy habits and patterns that work against your ability to create natural functional movement. If you are compensated in just one part of the equation then you are compensated in all. You will not get the correct result, much like the error of a math or physics equation, being off by one number somewhere in the calculations. Similarly with movement, you have to check and make sure movement is functional for good movement results. You, for instance, want to create a movement like a lunge, but can your body do it effectively after sitting at a desk eight hours a day?

It only takes one small change from misalignment to influence all the joints. It is the small change, so small, that it occurs unconsciously and painlessly, that has the most profound effect. Consciousness and mindfulness are the power to functioning better for movement, health, youth and vitality.

The Path to Pain:
Shallow breathing ⇨ Poor core stability ⇨ Poor spine stability ⇨ Poor posture ⇨ Misalignment/Compensation of joint stability ⇨ Poor joint mobility ⇨ Pain

Any of the above can start the cause of tension or pain.

Knee pain, for example, causes:
- asymmetry, shifting weight more to one side to squat, walk or run;
- a loss of range of motion caused by tension pulling, holding a joint in misalignment decreasing mobility that restricts movement;
- loss of strength in the knee, leg, hip and ankle; and
- hip imbalance through shifting to one side causing asymmetry.

Your body learns to function through compensation. Now you can see that when a joint is compensated, movement is compensated, as well as your awareness. Your range of motion becomes limited and dysfunctional. But as you improve your functional efficiency, you can improve range of motion, flexibility, strength and power more effectively instead of using a dysfunctional system.

Many people tell me it hurts when they run or when doing dead lifts, feeling that they can't perform those movements. But they can do those movements. The issues are not the movements but how they are moving in terms of mechanics, based on the functional operating system, to produce those movements. It's your alignment and stability that is weak, that disintegrates functional integrity from movement, which is how strain, pain and injury develop. **Function** is the result of the integrations that create **efficiency**. Strength training is all about efficiency.

Functional movement is the basic form your body uses to move:

- walking, running
- standing and sitting
- reaching to open a cabinet (arm extension)
- squatting
- lunging (for example, to pick a toy up off the floor)
- pushing, pulling
- bending over
- rotating your spine, your head

If the joints are not aligned and stable:

- muscle flexibility and range of motion are limited and creates muscle tension imbalance pulling joints into misalignment.
- energy transferring through the body is absorbed in the muscles and joints and not resolved through motion.
- the joints absorb the force individually that can wear away the joint and cause inflammation.
- muscles tighten and compensate movement because stability is not functioning.

The flexed spine runner, for example, will develop knee pain and other issues as well, for instance, cervical thoracic issues because the hips lack alignment and stability affecting the legs and spine. As he runs and generates force through the pounding of his feet on the ground, joint misalignments expose those joints and other joints to shear force, absorbing individual tension and shock. The joints lose stability and the surface area needed to distribute the impacts of force through the joints' alignment system. He thinks his knee is the problem, but it's not. It is the shift of misalignment that moves pressure and tension to other joints.

HOW DOES FUNCTION MOVE?

When you think of movement you probably think of a lunge, push-up, squat, etc. You are correct. They're all movements. But people rarely look at how they are functioning to move. Let's take a closer look at how joints communicate and function to move. The below chart will give you a better understanding about joint stability and mobility. The chart is excellent and is the work of FMS (Functional Movement Systems) and Gray Cook. I teach every joint has stability but every joint does not have mobility or have very limited mobility meaning it does not or should not move much.

Are your joints stable or mobile enough? (See Table 1 below.)
Movement Chart—Cause and Effect (by Gray Cook)

Table 1

Ankle	Mobility	Ankle **stabilizes and moves** the foot in running and walking.
Knee	Stability	Knee **stabilizes** your step to run, walk, lunge or jump.
Hip	Mobility	Hip creates **stability and mobility** to stand, run, jump, squat, and lunge.
Lumbar Spine	Stability	Lumbar **stabilizes** in bending, jumping, squatting, lunging, running and walking.
Thoracic Spine	Mobility	Thoracic **stabilizes** in a standing position and during running. It **moves** by rotating, bending side to side, hyperextending back and flexing forward.
Scapula	Stability	Scapula **stabilizes** the shoulder joint for shoulder mobility in pressing or pulling.
Shoulder Joint	Mobility	The shoulder joint **rotates** the shoulder and arm.
Lower Cervical	Stability	Lower cervical **stabilizes** turning your head side to side, tilting side to side and looking up and down.
Upper Cervical	Mobility	Upper cervical **stabilizes** an aligned position and **rotates and tilts** the head side to side and to look up and down.

The above chart represents joint-by-joint communication. I have added the lower cervical to the chart because this joint is needed to stabilize the upper cervical movements. Also note all mobility joints have stability as well.

Stability and mobility need to interact in order to create movement. Stability is a platform on which we produce mobility or movement. If on the one hand, every joint were stable, you would walk like Frankenstein's monster. But when standing, all the joints stabilize the body's alignment.

Table 1 shows where possible issues like compensation and dysfunction are located.

Runners, for example, who run fore-footed;

- lose mobility in the ankle because the calf muscles tighten.
- lose foot mobility stuck in a front anterior (forward) loaded position. The weight shift is on the toes or front of the foot.
- lose stability and contraction of the shin muscles (tibialis anterior).
- cannot squat or lunge well.

If the foot has a forward-weight shift (also called anterior-loaded), the ankle loses alignment and mobility. If the ankle joint is open, it cannot close, leaving it vulnerable to forces and loads when the foot/ankle steps to run or walk. It is similar to women who wear high heel shoes all the time and develop fractures or issues in their feet, which is very common today. The forward-weight shift disconnects the joint-to-joint communication. The knee loses alignment and stability because the ankle has lost its alignment and stability developing limited mobility. The foot now has limitations in movement. Usually the emphasis of the forward-weight shift of the foot causes the ankle to turn slightly outward, disrupting the tracking of the knee from the first two toes to over the four toes. The knee loses its alignment and may develop the mobility the ankle lost through this shift. The issue can be felt and compensated all the way up through the hip and spine. This compensation shifts through the whole body. To stop the compensation, fix the ankle by balancing muscle tension and running properly. This is one instance where all the joints of the body compensate and adjust.

When women stand on the floor out of their high heel shoes or when the fore-footed person puts their feet flat on the floor, they need to round the lumbar spine (hyperextension), sticking out their hips and glutes' to compensate for the stuck, tense muscles in the calves and for the compensation of the ankle losing alignment and stability. The joints need to shift and compensate because of the imbalanced muscular tension produced by joint misalignment and dysfunction. Remember, joint compensation happens naturally for our benefit. If you try to fix knee pain but the ankle does not develop alignment and stability of the whole foot and is the issue, the pain will continue or return and possibly damage more than one joint.

EXAMPLE: Use a mirror so you can see how this works. Lean forward on your toes. Let the heels come off the floor. When you lift the heels off the floor you will feel the hips tilting slightly. If not, lean forward into the toes more. When you lean forward more, to prevent yourself from falling, you will balance yourself by pushing your hips back, hyperextending the lumbar spine. If you have lumbar hyperextension, a forward hip tilt, when walking, running or moving forward you will have to shift the weight into the toes for walking to feel normal. If you have a posterior hip tilt, the spine rounds and the knees start to bend. In order to walk forward you shift the weight into the heel mid-foot and the foot flops forward to move. The alignment of the hips dictate the spines alignment, energy efficiency and the effectiveness of the pattern in which your will move, walk or run and how your feet will strike the floor. How you move and perform on the lowest level of movement like performing daily movement tasks is how you will function on a higher level of movement like strength training. It is alignment/misalignment that sends out the instructions of efficiency.

Don't try to justify range of motion first. Trying to move into greater ranges of motion produces injury. More is not better unless it is functional. Through alignment and posture, I see instantly why people move and run the way they do and why wear and tear, pain and strain develop. You can predict how a person will move based on the spine's postural alignment. I have trained wrestlers, judo athletes and others how to use their own alignment, as well as manipulate their opponents, to use leverage in technique. Make yourself functional and efficient and you will see movement patterns change for the best. As you change misalignment to alignment the respiratory, musculoskeletal and nervous systems integrate, become powerful and you will feel better and stronger with less fatigue.

HOW TO RUN FUNCTIONALLY AND EFFICENTLY

1. Hip alignment and stability is essential.

It facilitates posture, alignment and balanced muscular tension. The glutes strength produces stability and alignment for the hips. It transfers those forces to the abdominals and spine to stabilize. Nasal diaphragmatic breathing creates a force of pressure that is also stabilized by the abdominals and at the same time transfers stability to the spine. This whole process is the formation of the core. Each time you run, you strengthen the body to be that way. Train alignment, not misalignment.

2. The hips alignment initiates natural acceleration using gravity when you run.

When you run, keep the hips in alignment, not back. Don't initiate your step with your foot. Initiate your step with your hips. When you keep your hips in alignment, the foot will naturally step forward so you won't fall over. Try it. Lean your body forward. Lean forward a little bit more each time **without** pushing your hips back. Push your hips forward. When you don't push your hips back to prevent falling over and you push your hips forward, your leg/foot will kick out in front of you to prevent you from falling down. It's a reflex and you want to utilize and train this reflex when running. When you activate this reflex, stabilization is naturally activated. In doing this, you will increase the strength of the glutes and at the same time strengthen the hips to maintain alignment through running. This reflex produces efficient energy like letting the ball roll down the hill on it's own. The hips alignment enables the joints and muscles to function optimally and move the body properly with FE, developing balanced strength when running. On the contrary, with the hip tilt in misalignment, it does a very poor job at stabilizing and transferring forces, losing the mechanical advantage and natural acceleration, making running feel heavy, fatiguing and tiresome burdening each step. Weak alignment is not strong or prepared enough to handle forces. Running is all about how you transport your alignment; and what is in misalignment will produce strain, pain or injury, training strength imbalances. When you run with proper alignment, you strengthen that alignment to handle the forces generated. As the foot hits the floor, it creates the greatest amount of force and impact. So, hip alignment is needed to stabilize and transfer the impact and force properly, maintaining the mechanical advantage to naturally propel forward.

3.Most people compensate their hips and spine when they run. Producing a hip tilt affects the spine, especially when you are tired.

Try it. Walk with your hips back and spine hyperextended. Now move the hips in a forward position and walk. When the hips move into a forward position into better alignment, you will notice the connection of the foot stepping on the floor is stronger. Notice how each step is connected to the stabilization of the core and how the glutes' contraction is stronger. Notice when the hips are back, it feels heavier to lift the foot losing the natural reflex in your step. Notice when the hips are forward lifting the foot is easier, lighter and natural and the reflex is present to do it. The most important thing is having strong glutes' to maintain hip alignment to activate this connection. "Running with your hips" is a very small subtle running technique that provides so much power through alignment and leverage to run. It will feel like someone is pulling you forward with a rope. You will feel the legs naturally react with resiliency and springiness, activating the body's stability mechanisms. You will feel faster instantly but you have to train the motion for pace, strength and endurance.

4. Your foot strike is important.

The running alignment discussed above, will produce the heel to mid-foot strike through the big toe to maintain proper knee tracking. When you think of the heel strike, you don't need to land on the back of the heel with your toes pointing straight up into the air. It's about transferring the motion, like falling and rolling with ease. Landing on the whole foot with a slight heel strike creates transference through the foot and stimulates the glutes to stabilize. The heel has a reflex point for the glutes to contract. Therefore, in forefoot or mid-foot running, you lose that reflex and produce calf tension and inflexibility that changes the functional system. Forefoot running, stresses the ankle and knee more. It pulls the ankle joint open, reducing stability of the knee and weakness in the shin muscles, so of course forefoot running will feel easier if you trained yourself to do it. But that does not mean it is effective because it is easier. It means your body accepted the ankle and hip compensation.

Running with a very prominent heel strike will stress your heel. But using the heel to mid-foot strike has been proven to reduce the incidence of joint pain and is more energy efficient. It's about using the whole foot, not just the front or the back.

5.The best way to run is to make sure your joints are in alignment first.

Make sure muscles are not imbalanced creating tension and compensating a joint's position. Misalignment is the real threat and a problem to running and movement because of the repeated constant motion over time, increasing the pounds of pressure and creating wear and tear on joints, not using alignment to transfer and distribute forces. If you use the "lean forward method" that is taught in other books, it works. Anything that leans forward into gravity will accelerate, but using the reflex and movement from the hips, works more efficiently. Movement comes from the hips so you need to **lean** forward with your hips, not the spine. For example, if you stand up, squeeze your glutes' and shift the hips over your feet, you will feel the muscles on the bottom of your feet contract to stabilize and prevent you from falling over forward. This is the activation you want and need to initiate when running for natural acceleration. But if your hips lack alignment with a forward hip tilt and tight hip flexors and you **lean** the body forward under more hyperextension, or with a posterior hip tilt, tilted back, you lean the rounded spine forward, when you lean the misalignments forward, more force is applied to the misalignments. When the hips tilt forward or back, muscles in the lower back and thoracic spine for example, take a lot of shock abuse because of misalignment being disconnected from the structural alignment. **"Leaning forward" leans all the misalignments forward that produces strain.** Hip misalignment produces strength imbalance and training strength imbalance only strengthens the imbalance, training the body to stay that way, dysfunctional. Such a condition creates pain in the joints from poor posture and misalignment de-activating stability mechanisms. Poor stability of the hips, core and spine leads to other joints and muscles absorbing tension, developing aches and pains, instead of transferring energy (leverage). The lean forward concept is only half way there not taking into account structural alignment and how it functions.

6.If you run forefoot you may never experience problems, but you will when strength training.

If someone wants to squat, lunge, jump or shoulder press, etc., I have to make sure their alignment can produce range of motion safely and effectively first before adding any strength or power through a specific motion or program. The same goes for running. Joint alignment acts as a catalyst for symmetry in function. Form produces function. Function creates movement. Function is the most important step in the development of your movement because it will produce good habits for movement. If you are not aligned and out of balance, not functional, and asymmetrical, you need to eliminate compensation and misalignment to function first, move well and move more, not make it worse. If not corrected, as you move you will continue to disrupt the stability and mobility of the joints and the contraction and stretch of muscles in movement. Shifting function, shifts movement outcomes.

I can't tell you to run on your heel to mid-foot if your hips are tilted forward and spine is hyperextended. I can't tell you to run on your toes if your hips are tilted back and your spine is rounded forward. The compensated functional system your body is using just can't do it and the movement technique or pattern will not feel correct based on your physical and proprioception shift. You can only run the way your structural alignment is presently until you change misalignment to alignment. Running is not bad for you. It is your functional circuitry that is not good for running (remember, circle peg, square hole).

Chapter 4
Making the Unconscious Conscious
"Good habits formed at youth make all the difference."
"Quality is not an act, it is a habit." – Aristotle

HABITS: ADJUSTING, ADAPTING AND CHANGING

A habit is something you do from three to about a thousand times. But a thousand steps is really not a lot when you walk. Your brain formulates movement sequences it can move through and around using your present alignment/misalignment. The brain stores information for efficiency, which is how and why things become habitual. The longer you remain in misalignment moving around, the more tags and repetitions develop and create a habit training the neurological system. Every time you move, you program and train the system to operate that way. The neurological, neuromuscular system is formed around what is present. For example, each breath and step you take repetitively creates a tag in your proprioception system. It remembers what you did and how you did it, to do it again. The brain does not see good or bad; it is looking for the efficiency of movement to function through repetition. Doing ten good reps and doing ten bad reps is still just reps for the brain. What you train is what you produce. What you produce each day is your future in health, fitness or sport.

Positioning the body in a certain way will influence how you move. When a joint or muscle is in pain and you move into it a few times, it will cause you to alter and shift away from the pain. We change our position of alignment to be more comfortable. Gradually, other poor habits are generated from responding and repositioning the body to avoid feeling uncomfortable, aches and pains. You may wonder why other joints and muscles hurt and feel tight when you did nothing to cause them to hurt. It is because the joints were repositioned and don't work well in misalignment.

Unconscious actions change your function. Walking and talking on the cell phone, carrying your briefcase or a pocketbook with your arm up on the bag holding the strap, walking with a back pack on both shoulders or just one, sitting all day at a computer, standing writing on a chalkboard while shifting your weight and hips to one side or to one foot, or standing long periods of time shifting weight to one side. You create these misalignments and compensations that shift the body and your mind follows, saying, "OK, adjust, adapt and change," without you knowing you are creating a habit. These unconscious adaptations and adjustments affect alignment and movement health. Therefore, joints and muscles adjust and adapt to the situation.

Both the schoolteacher and the corporate office worker have good intentions about developing their health and strength. They don't realize that they are vulnerable to the demise of their own poor functional qualities. They need awareness about their work

51

positions to be efficient before participation. Just like cardiovascular testing, where heart rate and blood pressure are measured to make sure people are safe for cardiovascular exercise, movement requires the same understanding but with functional efficiency, breathing, alignment and stability first for safety before lifting weights and moving the body around. Ask yourself, when you train, do you just move mindlessly through ranges of motion when training; or are you training the functional mechanisms inside the range of motion to perform it well? What is happening in the range of motion is like the interior of a car motor. There are many mechanisms inside to make the motor perform to its capabilities. Much like the body moving, there are many functional mechanisms that make the body move and perform. If the mechanisms don't work well, then we lose ability and capability to develop and progress movement. Habits need to be positive to establish the underlying unconscious foundation to grow healthy and well, progressing what is good in life.

The littlest things have the greatest impact on energy, movement, thoughts and emotions, physical, non-physical, conscious and unconscious. Small misalignments get worse and worse and eventually lead to bigger issues like pain and injury. The whole system has to change.

CONSCIOUSNESS VS. UNCONSCIOUSNESS

Everything in our body communicates with each other: atoms, molecules, cells, muscles, joints, thoughts, emotions, etc. Breathing, stability, alignment, the posture and the joints all have an integrated unconscious neurological, neuromuscular connection. You can see how all the pathways affect each other, from breathing to alignment, to stability and movement. It is our job to get in touch with this communication by unfolding and unlocking each level of the unconscious mind to understand its power and consciously use it. Breathing better, joint alignment and movement are the physical external ways we can enter the portal into the connected unconsciousness. Becoming conscious and mindful to unconsciousness, changes habits and patterns to be functional and productive, telling us the secrets to health, youth and vitality.

Brainwashed by modern life, we become slaves to its connivance and mindless approaches, sitting in poor positions, compensating our posture and joints. You have to decide what kind of life you want. The sooner you understand this you can adjust and change for the better. There comes a time that you need to focus and start investing in your health, where you need to break the bad habits and conditioning creating limitations. When you break bad habits you break what was shackling health and vitality. You start activating health and what is associated and integrated with it. You open the door to its opportunities and rewards. But you have to focus on them. Each day you need to practice how you want your body and mind to develop for the next day to produce its true value.

By thinking and practicing that each day is another day you get younger instead of older, you take the first step to preserving the mind-body. Once you feel like you are getting older, each day becomes exactly that. What you feel is what your body believes and how your body responds. This is why I have you feel the examples, exercises and techniques in this book, to make them real. There is more power and understanding when you feel. When you feel you can transform. Transformation is the key to progression.

Consciousness is an awakening, an understanding of our potential or purpose. Unconsciousness is where all our potential is stored. But how do we open this locked box full of human potential? Once we become conscious and mindful we can change and express better outcomes. By practicing awareness, we develop mindfulness in the present rather than wandering the past or the future. Living in the past or trying to live in the future forgets all about maintaining the present. The present is where the past and future are activated. Being mindful changes our present, reversing the biological past and changing the future outcomes of our health. If we are mindful of our body, we can stop pain that developed in the past and prevent it from getting worse in the future. Transform the present to blueprint your future.

Breathing and Alignment Make the Unconscious Conscious.

UNDERSTANDING YOUR POTENTIAL

You have power in your body that is not fully used. People only use about 10 % of their potential, especially when breathing because they breathe shallowly through the mouth. They don't know how to breathe through the nose, and breathe just because it is automatic. Breathing and alignment help to unlock the unconscious powers of health movement, vitality and anti-aging, restoring and improving its function and mechanics. They are the gateways to health, youth, vitality and wellness, but yet they are unconscious, so underestimated and undertrained. The automatic functions, nasal diaphragmatic breathing and alignment adapt instantly throughout your day. The automatic functions have the most power because they are easily influenced to change for the good or the bad. Their purpose is survival, so they have a compensation mode that does not fail. They just switch to inefficiency without us knowing. Being mindful of them is the key.

The techniques in the next chapter of breathing will create the language your mind-body needs to translate the powers of the unconscious mind into consciousness potential. In order to search for powers in the unconscious mind, we need to search inside ourselves, striping away barriers and limitations, changing habits and understanding weakness to strengthen its functions. If you don't activate basic functions then you will not be conscious of other powers in your mind, establishing an inefficient potential. When a person learns nasal diaphragmatic breathing, they feel and see the differences in in health, fitness and sport, right away. They feel more functions and the ability to move better that were unconscious to them breathing through their mouth.

The sooner you become conscious, the better. It will prevent further damage and affliction. The more conscious you are of your body, the greater effect you can have on it. You can only create consciousness where you focus your mind. What are you focused on that takes precedence, pushing other things off the screen of awareness, especially your health? Strength is not always about what you need to do, sometimes it's about saying "no". It's about blocking the disruption and temptation of thought to infiltrate your choices. Don't always concentrate on strengthening your physical offense without strengthening your mental defense. There are many temptations and distractions that keep you from focusing on your health, youth, vitality and life. If you don't have quality, then everything will be inefficient, trickling down from the mind into the body, into the spirit and through life. The body becomes what you think and how you feel. A **mind** not focused on health and good choices leads to **physical (body)** diseases and disorders leading into **spiritual** discontent and unhappiness. As you become more conscious of your breathing, joints and alignment, you will notice changes in movement, awareness and energy that inspires your life.

What we transform today to feel younger, energetic and healthier is tomorrow's reward to become ageless and timeless.

Chapter 5
Your Breath Is Your Power
"Natural forces within us are the true healers of disease." – Hippocrates

The power of your breath will reverse pain, disease and prevent injury. It is the key to energy and vitality and is the powerful integration that produces the fountain of youth.

When people train, they fail to train strength without coordinating and integrating breathing into movement patterns, poses, exercises or even into life. Once your breathing is fatigued, limitations and compensations take place. The strength and size of your muscles do not matter when your breathing is fatigued. The person who can breathe well and move functionally and efficiently in their sport or performance has the most cardiovascular stamina, physical power and potential. Life, fitness and sport functions best when it is sustainable to perpetuate longevity and growth. Breathing powers everything from training, sports, health and energy to survival. It needs to be as functional and productive as possible, and can be the answer to being tired and fatigued as well as the limitation hindering progression.

The power of breathing is unconscious to us. It is automatic and involuntary. We don't think about it. Breathing just happens making us less aware to how it is functioning. Often we do not pay attention to whether we are breathing deep or shallow or through the nose or mouth. The only way to know is to be mindful of breathing, to feel it and train it in performance or life daily. What we feel is what truly activates mindfulness and its functions, not what we can consciously see. *Your breath is your power.* Breathing affects every aspect of the mind, body and spirit.

Life, health, youth, vitality, longevity, exercise and movement all depend on how you breathe. The failure to get breathing to regulate respiratory and cardiovascular demands first limits health and progression. When less efficient and effective, the body makes more effort through force and overtraining that nonetheless end up being subpar. Such results are primarily due to not training the diaphragm and breathing through the nose. This is a big issue in health and fitness today. People work and train harder than they can functionally breathe, hoping that it will make all their fitness dreams come true overnight. This is far from the truth. Once the breath becomes shallow during exercise, it's just a matter of time before you need to stop.

Let's look at running as an example. People try to run faster than they can actually breathe. The demand for oxygen becomes higher than the lungs can supply and the level of carbon dioxide (CO_2) is rising. The brain reacts by increasing the breathing rate to inhale more oxygen, hence, resorting to mouth breathing. If you can't maintain breathing through your nose and start sucking wind through your mouth, then you're running too hard, not meeting the level of demands produced by running—your training level is too high. Breathing through your mouth, sucking wind and panting causes your postural muscles to weaken reducing you to a rounded spine because of the lack of pressure and tension generated. When you except the compensation of breathing through the mouth, you create physical joint compensations and disrupt the levels of CO_2, leading to constriction in veins, arteries and muscles. Mouth breathing is neither an efficient nor qualitative way to breathe because of breathing into a smaller space (the top of the lungs) where there is limited capacity. Mouth breathing uses more breaths and energy per breath than one breath of nasal diaphragmatic breathing. If you run slower and focus on breathing through the nose using the diaphragm (tame the ego and don't assume that faster is better in the beginning), you will increase the amount of oxygen you take in and create stability for the joints, core and spine effectively, producing energy efficiency. When you run faster, you breathe faster but you need to train yourself to breathe in deeper and longer through the nose to regulate the demands being produced.

Over the years from training people how to strength train and run, most of them did not breathe correctly or well, providing the explanation of why they could not increase running endurance and why they were experiencing pain. After training and improving their breathing, all those people could run better, longer and experienced less fatigue. Even at rest they felt less fatigue in their recovery. They also started to become more mindful when running. They knew that when they felt fatigue to breathe deeper and to make sure that they were breathing through the nose to do it. This helped them run longer using their natural functional breathing pattern to manage their respiratory system effectively (relaxation mode) instead of breathing through the mouth. During running, if you are mindful of your breathing, you will prevent breathing through the mouth and the inhibition it produces against your performance.

With so much power, why is nasal diaphragmatic breathing underrated, undertrained and not practiced often by everyone? There are many breathing practices and methods. Some are simple and some are advanced in their training. The most important thing for you to do is always start simple and master simplicity to be functional. As you master simplicity you will build a strong foundation on which you can construct strength methods because it will provide structure, function and efficiency for progression. Without structure you can't make additions to support expansion. Without function you lose the integrations that produce movement, efficiency and its practicality. The loss of efficiency develops more strain and force. Forcing works against natural development. Therefore, you lose your functional ability

Remember: All training and performance is about training your breath.
You become what you train and train what you become.

BREATHE WITH YOUR NOSE, EAT WITH YOUR MOUTH

We are born breathing through the nose and eating with our mouth. Stress and the modern lifestyle have switched, compensated and evolved our breathing pattern to the mouth.

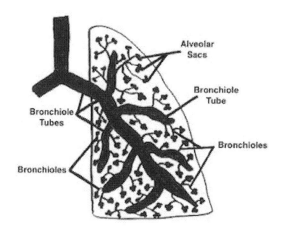

As you inhale air, it flows through the bronchial tubes and through the bronchioles (the smaller branches that ramify from the tubes) where the oxygenated air reaches the alveolar sacs.

As oxygen enters the sacs, it goes through the capillary where it then enters the blood.

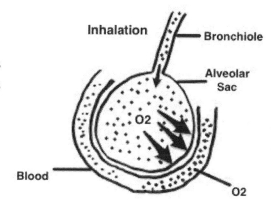

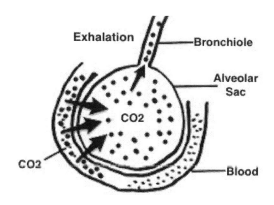

When you exhale and release the inhalation, it is just the exact opposite. CO_2 exits the blood via the capillary entering the alveolar sacs moving through the bronchioles, where CO_2's final path goes through the larger bronchial tubes and out of the nose or mouth.

How we breathe is crucial to our health, fitness and performance. There are two different ways to deliver oxygen to your lungs—mouth and nose. Mouth breathing is inhaling and exhaling through your mouth into the top of lungs. It is not very effective because the lungs are narrower at the top of the chest where there is less space and capacity in comparison to the lower area of the lungs. The top of the lungs does not expand like the bottom of the lungs because the diaphragm is not used effectively through mouth breathing. Using only a small amount of surface area in the upper lungs, in comparison to using a larger one in the lower lungs, produces strain that leads to dysfunctional breathing. When breathing through your mouth into a smaller surface area, it produces shorter and shallower breath's that increases the breathing rate. Increasing the breathing rate makes the heart work harder and faster to pump blood, producing a higher heart rate and blood pressure.

On the other hand, nasal diaphragmatic breathing (NDB) is inhaling through the nose. It contracts and flattens the diaphragm from its dome shape. NDB counteracts all the dysfunctional issues that mouth breathing produces. Which is why when people start to breathe through the nose, breathing problems and issues diminish and subside. When the diaphragm contracts, it pulls down the bottom of the lungs, increasing the size of the lungs about three times the size of the upper lungs. From the photos below, you can clearly see there is more surface area in the lower lungs than in the upper lungs containing vast amounts of alveoli to exchange O_2 and CO_2 in the bottom during inhalation. In one nasal diaphragmatic breath you can increase about 30 to 50 percent more O_2 and CO_2 exchanges than one mouth breath because of the diaphragm contracting and expanding the lungs, increasing the capacity in the lower lungs instantly. This results in breathing less, a lower heart rate and blood pressure, taking strain off the lungs and heart.

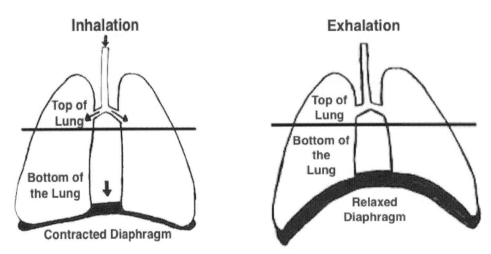

Lower area = more surface area = more exchanges = no strain, relaxed
Upper area = less surface area = less exchanges = strain, forcing the lung

WHY WE NEED CO₂

• **The amount of CO_2 that exits the lungs is very important because you do not want to clear all your CO_2 out of your body.** How we release it, through the nose, pursed lips or an open mouth, is pivotal. Breathing through the mouth produces an imbalance between O_2 and CO_2 quickly. You can breathe in and out more **liters of air quicker** in one breath through your mouth than your nose. But just because it's faster and does more, does not make it better. It produces dysfunction. Although you can inhale and exhale more air through your mouth, there is a very small percentage of O_2 that gets inhaled and perfused because mouth breathing causes CO_2 levels to remain low. When you exhale through the mouth it release to much CO_2 than the nose does, producing imbalance. The nose is a better system to control airflow.

• **Inhaling as much air as you can, taking in many deep breaths through your mouth, does not mean you are increasing the amount of O_2 in your body.** It is the exact opposite. If CO_2 levels are low in the blood then O_2 will not be released or inhaled. If your body does not need oxygen or it is not exchanged properly then it is just a wasted breath. A wasted breath consumes energy and produces strain on the heart. Breathing through the mouth at rest or during exercise, exhales too much CO_2 at one time, making the levels drop too quickly, creating O_2 deficit and deficiency. It is a big reason why muscles get tight and constricted at rest, during exercise, fitness and sports performance because of poor regulation. It is a big reason why fatigue sets in quicker because blood flow is constricted. The large amounts of CO_2 exhaled through the mouth produces an alkaline condition in the blood that constricts arteries and veins affecting the brain and the heart as well as muscles decreasing the cardiovascular and musculoskeletal systems performance. When CO_2 levels fall, O_2 is held and not released from the blood. It is why the mouth is not a functional way to breathe at all. This is one perfect example of how the respiratory dysfunction strains the cardiovascular, musculoskeletal and neurological systems. Inhaling through the nose creates dilation where as inhaling through the mouth creates constriction.

• **CO_2 is the primary factor for your breathing rate to increase or decrease and instructs the blood what to do with O_2.** There are receptors (chemoreceptors) in the veins and arteries that send information to the brain about CO_2 levels in the blood. As CO_2 levels rise, it releases stored O_2 from hemoglobin in the blood and travels to cells and muscles that need it. But when CO_2 is low, O_2 is not released from hemoglobin, the blood, because it is not needed. CO_2 is the main factor that releases O_2 at rest and during exercise. For this reason, CO_2 is a signal calling for O_2, showing work was produced and more O_2 is required. The blood does not give up O_2 as freely as you think. Your blood holds O_2 until it really needs to release it, until there is an affinity, an attraction, a need for it, from metabolic cellular reactions at rest to exercise when CO_2 levels rise rapidly because of working muscles and cells. It is a survival mechanism for the body. But like I just said, breathing through the mouth makes this process dysfunctional because of **poor breathing mechanics**.

• **CO_2 is more easily released from the body than O_2 perfusion.** O_2 needs the proper conditions to enter the capillary. CO_2 is a byproduct of cellular metabolism that is released from the body naturally. It has a higher and quicker rate of release because it does not require anything for it to be released, just exhaling. No attraction, no affinity is needed. We simply create breathing issues by breathing through our mouth, creating constantly low CO_2 levels. If the same were true for O_2 to be used and taken in so easily, we would be highly oxygenated people with high VO_2 levels, volume of oxygen. But unfortunately, it's not the same. Your mouth is just a secondary emergency way to breathe and used to eat. Controlling CO_2 through how we breathe is the key to O_2 utilization.

• **The body maintains a certain level of O_2 and CO_2 in the alveoli (100mm/hg O_2) (40 mm/hg CO_2) during a resting state.** The objective of nasal diaphragmatic breathing at rest is to produce more **exchanges** of O_2 and CO_2, like building a bigger motor and gas tank that can utilize more energy. Therefore, you breathe less per minute making the heart more efficient to beat less per minute because of **more exchanges**. On the contrary, breathing through the mouth makes the lungs work harder increasing the breathing rate per minute (hyperventilating) directly increasing the heart rate per minute. The heart has to pump harder and more, increasing the rates per minute because of O_2 deprivation to the heart, muscles, etc. It's not about clearing all your CO_2 because you need it! How you breathe is the difference between health and disease, vitality and fatigue, feeling young or old.

• **As oxygen demands increase during exercise, we need to meet those demands.** For this reason, by taking deeper, longer and fewer inhalations through the nostrils, we can neutralize the demand for oxygen more effectively, without strain, into the bigger more abundant space of the lower lungs, using the whole lungs, where more alveolar sacs are present, maximizing volume and performance. If you want this process to really be effective, increase the amount of capillaries and mitochondria's in your muscles as well, exactly what exercise does. This will make your body much more effective at utilizing O_2 during exercise and in a resting state.

• **Society has been misled into thinking that CO_2 is toxic and bad for you, when it is actually the opposite.** CO_2 is an important gas because it is a natural vasodilator. In the nasal passages there is a gas called nitric oxide (NO) that is produced naturally. In an abstract according to PubMed.gov, *Nitric oxide and the Paranasal Sinuses*, nitric oxide produces vasodilation, a natural dilating gas that expands the bronchial tubes and bronchioles, making it easier for more air to pass delivering oxygen to the blood. NO also acts as an antimicrobial that filters the air in your nose preventing bacteria and pollutants from entering your body. Breathing through the nose keeps the presence of CO_2 in the airflow, at a minimal level, to maintain dilation. This is one significant quality that can only be achieved from nasal breathing and can solve many physical ailments by retraining the breathing process.

• **Vasodilation means that veins and arteries expand, stay open, which is what CO_2 promotes, not constriction.** This means the arteries and veins dilate for O_2 to be released in the areas of **high CO_2 concentrations**, where it is needed most. CO_2 relaxes muscles, stimulates nerves, especially to the brain, and reduces inflammation in joints and the body because of its dilation qualities. So, when CO_2 is produced it signals and prepares the path for O_2. For example, when **CO_2 is high**, O_2 will be released from the blood easily to balance an acidic environment of CO_2 where CO_2 facilitates the process of vasodilation for O_2 delivery. When **CO_2 is low**, blood vessels constrict (vasoconstriction) and less O_2 is released (Bhor Effect) because there is no affinity (attraction) or need for it. If **CO_2 is low**, vasoconstriction affects the brain, organs, muscles, arteries, veins and the systemic. Vasoconstriction produces strain on the lungs, heart, arteries and veins affecting the function, integration and dynamics of the respiratory and cardiovascular systems. That is the beauty of CO_2's power, having the affinity to prepare and attract O_2. What depends on the success to maintain the ability to intake and release O_2 properly is based on CO_2 levels. This is especially important to sustain energy, health and vitality. It is extremely important for sports performance to keep veins and arteries under vasodilation to maintain energy and power.

Example: Make sure you are sitting down. Read first so you will understand the effects. Inhale and exhale through your mouth 5 to 8 times deeply. Wait for about one minute and you will start to feel lightheaded from mouth breathing within that minute. Relax for a few minutes reset and come back to focus. Now perform the same number of repetitions keeping the mouth closed and only breathing through the nose 5 to 8 times the same way. You will notice the nose has more control over the flow of air than the mouth. The flow of air through the mouth is erratic and too much, that leads too expelling too much CO_2. The reason you felt lightheaded from mouth breathing is because the mouth expels too much CO_2 at one time. The nose provides regulation. When CO_2 levels fall, O_2 stays bounded and not released by the blood producing an alkaline state in the blood constricting veins and arteries leading to lightheadedness. You may have felt a little light

61

in the head from the nasal breathing but not as much or as high in comparison to mouth breathing. You felt that little bit of lightheadedness in nasal breathing because your breathing is not trained.

UNCONSCIOUS EFFECTS OF POOR BREATHING MECHANICS

Many situations in life can change how we breathe from the nose to mouth from deep to shallow; like being sick with fever, flu, stress, depression, fear, sitting too much, fatigue, not sleeping well, being sedentary or from living the modern lifestyle. At some point poor breathing dynamics take over to imbalance life, physical health, create joint inflammation, increase blood pressure, and produce muscle pain and tension. We allow it to happen and train it into our system to adapt and function with it in everyday life. The problems that arise from breathing through your mouth and shallow breathing are: asthma, headaches, tight muscles (especially in the neck and back), inflexibility, fatigue, decreased cardiovascular capacity, increased heart rate, increased blood pressure, lung infections etc. On the contrary, there are a few very important and crucial qualities that can be attained from breathing through the nose and not the mouth that can prevent the problems associated above.

Over time, it is the cardiovascular issues like increased heart rate and blood pressure that eventually become cardiovascular diseases, trickling down, producing other imbalances, diseases and disorders in the body. There's no buffer or control from breathing to establish the balance and function of pressure, tension and exchanges, so force and strain make the heart work harder. Doctors do not teach you how to breathe. They inspire and recommend you to exercise. It's up to you to make the unconscious breathing pattern conscious by using it. As you can see, breathing affects the respiratory system that affects the cardiovascular system's responses, impacting the musculoskeletal and central nervous systems. Such is the power of breathing and all the unconscious systems' connections. Changing how you breathe will change how you feel and how you move. It will bring benefit and reward instantly because your breathing can adapt and adjust in an instant. You have the power to make the unconscious conscious.

You now know how you are breathing and understand its power and capacity to change your life and health. Breath is your life force. It's your power. Its power is based on simplicity. You already breathe—inhale and exhale. The only adjustment you need is to breathe through the nose and train your breath. The challenge is not to fall into the bad habit of mouth breathing. Stay mindful of your breath and keep stress and emotions in check. What you are mindful of will start to construct your life. This is the reason we need to be aware of breathing, alignment and the things we eat and do in the moment, because they are going to construct our future habits and health. *Being mindful of your breath gives you control and power over your life.* Awareness and consciousness of the breathing pattern is a must. Losing awareness of the breathing pattern compensates instantly. Remember, it is an automatic function with a failsafe switch. Be conscious to breathe to produce the circuitry for health and exercise. Mindfulness is the key.

BREATHING IN MOVEMENT

When you know you are going to exert force to jump, sprint, tackle, push or pull, you generate pressure through breathing to be released into the exertion of movement or to stabilize the movement. It all depends on the movement you are performing. The idea is to maintain abdominal tension naturally, as you breathe. Breathing in movement is like stretching a rubber band then letting it go to release it's energy. Remember, *"Inhalation encourages the contraction of most muscles and exhalation encourages their relaxation."* (Travell and Simons). Since the body can move and exert force in many different directions, breathing and exertion depends on the movement and direction. If you don't have pressure and tension then you won't generate force and power. Dr. Stuart McGill refers to this as *"bracing breath"* He says, *"bracing breath transfers to the spine and muscles throughout the body."* The more intra-abdominal pressure produced from nasal diaphragmatic breathing, the more tension the abdominals and the core will have that can be transferred through movement; pressing, throwing, jumping, running, etc. It is the reason why breathing transfers strength through and to muscles. Mouth breathers cannot do this effective. They don't have a regulated breathing pattern that is functional or progressive. Mouth breathing does not produce the intra-abdominal pressure needed to produce abdominal tension and nor has maximal power to be release in movement.

When I teach clients to breathe, I teach them a few different ways to breathe during movement. One way is inhaling and exhaling through the nose. The second way is inhaling through the nose and exhaling through pursed lips. This second way of breathing releases CO_2 at a regulated rate and not too much so quickly like open mouth breathing does. When you exhale using pursed lips, it is like blowing through a straw. There is a reflex in the exhalation of air through pursed lips that makes the abdominals tense and the core stabilize. Try it! Inhale through your nose for 3 seconds and exhale pushing the air through pursed lips, like blowing through a straw. The harder you push the air through pursed lips, the more the abdominals produce isometric contraction. I have taught this method to many students, clients and athletes because it is extremely beneficial to use during sports, strength training and running to maximize performance, power and energy. It is a very multi useful and powerful way to breathe. Increasing the power of your breathing enhances abdominal tension. Enhancing abdominal tension augments strength. Breathing properly maximizes and conserves energy. Many understand the reasons for their fatigue now, having to push and force through their exercises in the past. However, it is unnecessary to force exercise and strength if you are breathing correctly in your training, sustaining the needs for oxygen, pressure and tension to move. If you feel tired, check how you are breathing. Breathing needs to be normal and regular not forced and compensated. Your breath works with alignment and movement in an integrated and coordinated process, especially with stability. The joints and spine have a kinetic link and an unconscious neuromuscular connection to breathing. If you are breathing through the mouth then the core will not develop and the spine will not have connectivity producing flexion (rounding forward) and poor stability. How you breathe influences posture and joint alignment.

The breathing techniques in this book will help you develop a functional breathing pattern that institutes good health and creates a stable core to transfer through mobility and movement. Sometimes it's a pace like when running and sometimes it's for more tension to move deeper into a strength pattern or to resolve movement. Knowing, training and practicing breathing will put you on top of the competition. I have taught many people, including athletes, to dramatically improve their movements and sport. In rugby, I taught and trained players how to develop pressure and tension through breathing, coordinating it with their playing techniques to move the ruck, tackle and sprint. In judo, I taught and trained players how to throw more powerfully. For rowers, I taught them how to create a powerful endurance tank of energy. I have taught clients to breathe better from the improvement of posture to the development of the core. It is not necessary to learn yoga to improve your breathing. Yoga is a form of exercise that works with breathing. All forms of exercise should work with breathing first, alignment and stability second and movement third. It is the integration of the three that creates motion, functional efficiency and work as a catalyst setting the platform for a movement pattern and it's power: to throw, ruck, squat or lunge, etc. If you're not breathing correctly, you're not going to produce stability in the core and the pressure needed to produce tension for the abdominals, especially if you breathe into the chest. You cannot create and manipulate the core as a fulcrum to stabilize the spine and move powerfully. If you are not stable, then balance, coordination and transference of movement is difficult. Imagine jumping off a dock into the water. Now imagine jumping into the water off a canoe. There is a big power difference between the two due to the stability of the platform in which you jump to coordinate the power to move. Breathing is the timing chain to coordinate and synchronize all functions in movement patterns, exercises and poses.

When you perform movement patterns and poses, think about how your breathing can best establish pressure for abdominal tension in the pattern or pose. This is essential when increasing the intensity of a movement or adding weight. The breath needs to be trained into movement through repetition, building the strength of the diaphragm to contract and relax, to be resilient. It matters how you breathe to the core in movement, not how much weight you can move physically. That comes later.

When I work on breathing with someone, I always ask: What sensations do you now feel? The answer I always get is, "I feel light and more upright." When posture is strong and balanced, you feel less tension and less gravity pulling on you, thus making you feel lighter and more energetic in your body, balancing energy. Alignment and stability thus communicates harmony to joints and muscles. It prevents misalignment and instability from making adjustments in the body that use so much energy to maintain imbalance. How we respond to gravity's pull is what forms our proprioception system. Before you learn the breathing exercises find out if you are a chest or abdominal breather.

Chest or Abdominal Breathing Test

- Lie down on your back. Place your hands on your chest and abdomen.
- Start to breathe.
- Feel which rise's first—the chest or abdominals.

It is desirable to have the abdominals react and slightly rise first to fill the bottom of the lungs and have air travel up to the chest. Breathing into the chest cannot pull air down into the bottom of the lungs. You are therefore not utilizing full capacity of the lungs because you are not using the diaphragm.

A quick correction is to lie on your stomach and clasp your fingers together. Place your forehead on the clasped fingers and breathe into the stomach through your nose. The floor will give pressure to the abdominals, providing stimulation to the diaphragm. Crocodile breathing is a good way to correct and learn how to breathe into the abdomen. It's also very relaxing.

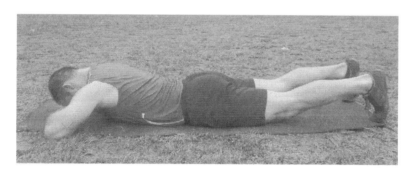

Another correction is to clasp your fingers together and place them on your stomach over the navel in a seated or standing position. Breathe in through the nose and place pressure on the abdominals by pushing the clasped hands into the abdominals as you inhale. As you push the hands on the abdominals, they will create tension. Use the breath to provide pressure as a foundation behind the abdominals. At the same time, pull your elbows into the ribcage. You will feel the lats and back muscles contract along with the abdominal tension and the inhalation.

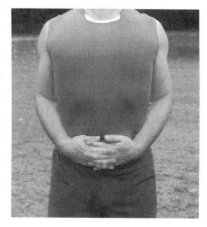

USING THE DIAPHRGAM FOR RUNNING AND TRAINING

Many people begin their fitness program by jumping on a cardiovascular machine, watching TV and running like robots. They use machines to produce muscular strength without using their breath in any way integrated to movement. Being attuned to how the body moves and feels is important, but it requires awareness. Being mindful of your breathing during exercise, you can take its cues to help you regulate heart rate, be more efficient and more effective. Learning to breathe through the nose prevents the hearts beats per minute from spiking too high that can extend endurance. When strength training, it connects us to the musculoskeletal system to maximize strength production. Breathing can be trained and controlled to make changes at an instant.

During an exercise like running (when tension builds) it is preferable to control breathing—to establish pace, rhythm and take fewer deeper and longer breaths using the diaphragm, not more. Using nasal diaphragmatic breathing during running is more suitable for energy conservation as well. You need to take cues on when to inhale and exhale to train and regulate your breathing pattern. In the beginning, you will probably find your breathing rhythm is a bit erratic. Just keep focusing on inhaling through the nose and relax your breathing. You can also run inhaling through the nose and exhaling through pursed lips as well. You can adjust the breathing pattern to inhale and exhale through your nose or exhale through the pursed lips, to prevent the release of too much CO_2 and to maintain abdominal pressure. As you train your running, you will notice your breathing starts to get deeper and longer and will find slight pauses when breathing, taking less breaths per minute and becoming more relaxed. More relaxed means the respiratory system is not straining and is performing functionally. Nasal diaphragmatic breathing promotes relaxation of the nervous system to synchronize the respiratory and cardiovascular systems performance optimally. Once you have established the rhythm and control of your breathing, you can synchronize the breathing with your foot strike. This is where you will economize and conserve energy more efficiently. But you need the breathing foundation first.

When running, **the inhalation** produces the contraction of the diaphragm to increase the volume of oxygen and stabilize the core and all the postural muscles to keep the torso stable and aligned to transfer forces. In the same breath, it facilitates and supports muscular contractions to maintain joint alignment and stability overall through your foot strike. Therefore, inhalation activates the diaphragm that produces the pressure for the core and tension for the abdominals, to stabilize the forces generated through the foot strike. The secret to breathing and running is to inhale longer and deeper through the nose using the diaphragm for more strides and exhaling for less. This helps to maintain pressure and stability in the core. You need to have the greatest amount of stability and optimal joint alignment at the time of impact, not less. You always need to have pressure to maintain stability and tension transference. When you run, for example, try inhaling through your nose for 6 running steps or 4 seconds and then exhale through your nose for 3 running steps or 2 seconds. Continue this technique through your running. You can always adjust the ratio for yourself personally. It is more about what gives you the most control in the beginning and expanding upon that foundation for progression. You don't have to be stuck to the numbers the whole time. You have to train the process. You have to listen to what the body needs at the time of performance. Learn to adjust your running around your breathing. If you need to run slower, run slower and train the natural functional breathing process. If you don't, you will compensate progression. Train utilizing the lower lung to develop a higher volume of oxygen, in turn running will develop capillaries and mitochondria that also improve the efficiency and effectiveness of oxygen utilization. Not listening can lead you down a different path creating fatigue because you are trying to do more than the system can handle at that time.

In strength training, you need to control and train your breathing to produce more stability through repetitions. You need to activate the core through the inhalation of the nose to produce a high stabilizing pressure needed through movement because of adding weights and load. The high stabilizing pressure makes you stronger instantly because it stimulates the nervous and neuromuscular system's amplitude and electrical frequency. When you increase pressure, you increase tension and that is what stimulates the nervous system's circuitry to transmit power through the musculoskeletal system to perform. When you exhale you exhale through pursed lips that activates the reflex for the abdominals to stabilize that facilitates spine stability. How you breathe is important in repetition for timing, coordination and synchronization. Most people develop subpar strength and potential because they only train the musculoskeletal system not the respiratory or nervous systems properly. The nervous system is what produces strength and power in the musculoskeletal system. But like anything, you need to practice and use the proper programing to facilitate the best results. When you stop practicing breathing techniques you lose power much like when you stop strength training, you lose some strength. It needs to be a daily practice.

As you perform strength programs or running with poor breathing mechanics, the loss of (inhalation) stability gets transferred to the joints through motion. Losing stability is like losing the shock absorbers on your car. They can't diffuse and transfer the forces applied and generated to and through the whole body. Instead, force gets stuck and absorbed by the joints and muscles individually, producing pain or strain. As you continue to train with poor breathing technique, you are transferring and training the compensations and inefficiency through the system. Training the process of nasal diaphragmatic breathing is important because each process triggers the next. Inhaling through the nose triggers the diaphragm to pull down the bottom of the lungs to increase the space and capacity for more oxygen volume. At the same time, the inhalation produces the pressure and stability for the core and spine, triggering the nervous systems power. Without using the breath as the trigger, the integration of the cardiovascular, nervous and musculoskeletal systems lead to less effective results. Without inhaling through the nose first, the sequence will be compensated. I have observed notable improvements in clients' strength, range of motion and mobility as they learn how breathing and stability work together. Nasal diaphragmatic breathing is therefore the missing piece to complete the puzzle of increased performance, fitness, vitality and health for longevity.

Nasal Breathing	Mouth Breathing
Learned as a baby.	Learned as an adult.
Longer, deeper breaths, lower breathing rate.	Shorter, quicker, erratic faster breathing rate.
Lower heart rate and blood pressure.	Higher heart rate and blood pressure.
Uses the diaphragm.	Does not use diaphragm.
Breathes into the lower lungs for vast amount of exchanges increasing volume of oxygen and decreasing the amount of breathes per minute.	Breathes into the upper lungs for minimal amount of exchanges decreasing the volume of oxygen and increasing breaths per minute.
Produces pressure to strengthen the core, abdominals and the posture and spine.	Cannot do.
Uses Nitric Oxide.	Cannot do.
Balances O2 and CO2 exchange.	Offsets the balance.
Parasympathetic (Slow).	Sympathetic (Rapid and Fast).

ONE-MINUTE BREATHING TEST

WARNING: If you find any of the breathing exercises difficult and challenging, never hold your breath unless you have been trained to do so first. You have to learn to adapt and adjust to the exchange of O_2 and CO_2 as well as the pressure. Holding your breath is detrimental if you are not trained to do so and have respiratory or cardiovascular issues.

Let's see how many breaths you take in one minute. Just breathe normally for one minute. Use your everyday breath, that is, don't inhale so your shoulders rise and struggle to get the last bit of air in to perform fewer breaths in the time. If you are a mouth breather then breathe through you mouth. If you breathe rapidly, then do it for the test or you will be missing the point here. If you don't know what is dysfunctional, you will not know how to advance.

- One breath is both an inhalation and an exhalation.
- Breathe how you breathe without strain in your breath.

Remember this is practice and training. It does not mean you have to walk around trying to breathe for three breaths a minute normally, like in your practice. Before you begin, take your heart rate for one minute and your blood pressure if you have the capability. Chart your progress using breaths per minute and heart rate. Retest after every three to five faithful practice days.

Breaths in one minute, the results from the one-minute test:
Excellent: 3 breaths or less per minute
Good: 3 to 12 breaths per minute
Average/ Normal: 12 to 18 breaths per minute
Poor: 18 or more breaths per minute

I take two and a half to three breaths a minute in my **breathing practice, my training.** My resting heart rate is 48. My first breath is 22 seconds, the second is 25, and I start the third breath at 47 seconds. When I breathe **normally at rest** for the one-minute test, I breathe six breaths per minute. The test is not the training. I test for six breaths with normal breathing in one minute without focusing on trying to inhale deeper and exhale slower. I train and practice using two and a half to three breaths per minute, concentrating on control to relax, slowly inhaling and slowly exhaling to create capacity, volume, strength and pressure. The breathing practice, the training, helps my breaths per minute become lower at rest. When time gets longer for breathing, it is good. It is becoming more efficient.

As you become trained, you don't need to breathe as much and you breathe and will take pauses before the next breath through the nose. Try it. Sit down. Take a deep breath through the nose at pace, not too fast, can be slow. Now, exhale it out fully through the nose. Now notice when you needed to take the next breath? It was not instantly. Therefore, you are not breathing in and out constantly because the body does not require another breath just yet, especially at rest. This is nasal diaphragmatic breathing using more surface area in the lungs effectively for more O_2 and CO_2 exchanges with less breaths, not more breaths, maintaining the balance. Nasal diaphragmatic breathing produces a stronger and higher-pressure gradient than the mouth that affects the control, inhalation and exhalation. Like I said before, you can inhale and exhale more air breathing through the mouth but it is not functional and has less control. Mouth breathing is **not hardwired** to utilize and regulate O_2 and CO_2 properly. You are using less surface area breathing into the top of the lungs with too much airflow and strain that cannot perform the exchanges functionally.

It has been proven that most people who are mouth breathers breathe more than 12 times a minute, and may suffer from COPD, asthma or allergies. It has been scientifically proven that heart disease is linked to shortness of breath and oxygen deprivation to the heart from mouth breathing. Breathing through the mouth has a high correlation with high blood pressure. It also has a high link with anxiety, depression, stress, tension and many emotional disorders.

THE BREATHING EXERCISES: ACTIVATING THE DIAPHRAGM

When most people exercise, run or perform strength training, one of the reasons for their fatigue is because they are not breathing properly. This impacts the integration between the systems, affecting endurance, strength, power output and results.

There are many different ways to breathe. The two types I focus on work with nasal diaphragmatic breathing. The first is breathing in and out of the nose that is required for more repetitive aerobic type of movements like running. The second type of breathing is breathing in through the nose and hissing the air out the mouth with pursed lips that you will use in this book. The second type of breathing is used for movement patterns and strength training because you need to maintain pressure in the core when moving weights around, stretching muscles and moving joints in different angles and directions to maintain stability. Exhaling through pursed lips does this perfectly. Bracing breath (pursed lips) maintains a higher level of power and stability. The hiss out of the mouth (pursed lips) activates the abdominal stability. Combining both gives you a powerful combination in sports like rugby, hockey, martial arts, judo, football, etc. The hiss is also effective when running, especially for speed. What's most important is that you inhale through the nose and exhale your air through minimal space like the nose or pursed lips to retain air and pressure. All in all, it depends on what is more comfortable for you. How fast you release the exhalation is what makes the difference: pausing or slightly holding depends on the activity at hand. As you develop this breathing pump, the abdominals, diaphragm and lungs become stronger and so does your stability.

Making Contact with the Diaphragm – Learning to Inhale

- Sit up straight or stand. Try to keep the shoulders back. The shoulders will create tension on the spine's postural alignment producing connectivity for the abdominals to react.
- Breathe in through your nose.
- As you breathe in, keep the abdominals tight to prevent the stomach from distending. **You will feel the tension in the abdominals, ribcage and up the spine when you don't push the stomach out.** This technique will strengthen your lungs, the diaphragm, the abdominals, the core and postural muscles, producing stability between the core and spine, all at the same time. You are not sucking in your stomach. You are tensing and creating a wall in the abdominals that tightens from the inhalation.
- Create pressure, as far as you are comfortable. Keep the abdominals

tight producing a wall of tension matching the breath's pressure coming in.
- Exhale at any pace you want for now through the nose or pursed lips. Just concentrate on inhaling, producing pressure for abdominals to create a wall of tension for a strong diaphragmatic contraction. Let the abdominals and breath go, and feel the breath naturally exhale.
- Practice for 10 breaths

Bracing the abdominals with the inhale starts to develop the core. If you distend your stomach when you inhale, you will not feel the pressure and tension in the core, spine and the rib cage. If you have a rounded spine, slouched and rounded shoulders, try to sit up straight with good posture and pull the shoulders back as you do the breathing exercises. Go slow. When your posture is poor the diaphragm and other muscles in that area are probably restricted.

(Note: Many programs practice stomach distention, but such a practice lacks the ability to transfer tension. Sucking the abdominals in makes the spine round.)

The Hiss: Learning to Exhale
- Breathe in through the nose to the abdominals with abdominal bracing tension.
- Keep your lips pursed.
- Now instead of letting the breath, the abdominal tension go like the first technique, keep the abdominals tight and push the air through pursed lips. It should feel like blowing slowly through a straw. As you do this, the abdominals will stay tight automatically from the reflex. The more your mouth is open the less pressure and the less tension the abdominals produce with no reflex. Let it happen naturally right now.
- You will feel a belt forming around the hips and back. As you hiss you will feel the pressure build up strengthening the lungs.
- Don't worry about breathing at full capacity here. Inhale for about 3 to 5 seconds. Tighten the abdominals around the inhalation. Then, exhale with pursed lips activating the abdominals isometric contraction. Practice for 10 breaths, inhaling and exhaling. Build up to long inhalations and exhalations to train the lungs.

Breath, stability and pressure create transference of tension and pressure through the body radiating strength and stability through the joints and muscles (musculoskeletal and neuromuscular systems) for strong movements. Practice this exercise regularly at rest to strengthen your lungs and incorporate it into you training programs. It will help to improve performance in running or any other activity. Inhale to contract and stabilize. Exhale to relax for more motion and to release the tension for power in the movement.

Below are breathing exercises to expand your functionality.

Lung Resiliency
Breathe in slowly and deeply. Exhale slowly to develop breathing capacity, strength, endurance and stamina.

- Stand or sit comfortably.
- As you breathe in through your nose, tighten your abdominals to match the breath you are slowly inhaling. The deeper you breathe, the tighter you want to make the abdominals. Feel like a balloon is filling up inside your stomach but your stomach is not distending.
- Try to breathe into the lower abdominal basin below your navel.
- As you tighten the abdominals more, you will feel the diaphragm tighten more pulling down.
- Keep the abdominals tight, so as you breathe, pressure and tension will cover a greater surface area. Practice slowly to learn how to train and maintain this space and pressure.
- To strengthen your breathing, breathe in deeper and tighten the abdominals more to increase the power of the breath coming in. It is like hooking your two index fingers and trying to pull them apart, isometrically increasing the tension.
- Don't push out your stomach.
- Actively exhale by hissing the air out through pursed lips. Try to maintain control of the pressure when exhaling. Depending on how hard you push your air out and how tight the lips are makes the abdominals tighten more or for less.
- Repeat 5 to10 times.

If you breathe out of an open mouth, you will not maintain pressure or tension. If you need to breathe out of the mouth, then breathe. But resist the temptation to open your mouth. **Breathe if you need to and never force it!**

The Hiss Keeps the Abdominals Pressurized.
- An open mouth decreases abdominal pressure.
- A slightly open mouth trains you to retain pressure.
- A closed mouth holds pressure.

When running you may use softer pursed lips and during strength use a tighter pursed lip to produce more pressure.

Stamina – Ladder Breaths

You can start breathing in for a count of 5 seconds and then exhale for a count of 5 seconds, then 6 and 6, 7 and 7, 8 and 8, 9 and 9, 10 and 10. Then work your way back down to 5. Choose a time that is comfortable for you. Try to do it for 3 to 5 minutes. It is easy to do just a few times. You need to build up the strength of your breathing for stamina and endurance. You can also breathe in for 5 seconds and breathe out slowly for 8 seconds. Always try to do it for a given amount of incremental time. Your breath will get stronger and you will be learning control.

CAUTION: Do not strain or force breathing. Stop if it feels uncomfortable. If you have issues with your lungs and heart, seek your doctor's advice first before proceeding with the exercises.

Inhaling slowly will exercise the diaphragm's contraction, increase the capacity of VO_2 and develop the lungs' pressure system. Slowly exhaling will eccentrically strengthen the diaphragm and train the lung's pressure system, developing endurance and resiliency. Just like muscles, you want the lungs to be resilient as well. You ultimately want to train your lungs to take fewer breaths per minute at rest, during exercise, running and training by increasing the length of your breath to increase VO_2 and core stability at the same time. Such efficiency leads to highly effective conditioning. You have to imagine that the heart rate, blood pressure and breathing are gauges for the body. If breathing is not efficient, when it is belabored, the gauges will adjust for those responses.

Use control and direction of the breath when breathing. Believe it or not, just because you breathe does not mean you breathe evenly to the core. People breathe more into one side than the other, which develops breathing asymmetry and core strength imbalance. This imbalance can affect the stability of the abdominals and that projects spinal misalignments, shoulder issues, neck issues and poor posture, resulting in structural asymmetry. When structural asymmetry is present it leads to dysfunctional movement. As you breathe, use your fingers to press into the right and left sides of the abdominals to feel for strength asymmetries. You will feel a spot a litter softer than the rest of the abdominal area. When you find the softer spot, press your fingers into the spot and breathe into your fingers pressure and feel the abdominals tighten like other spots. The breath helps to align the spine from the sacrum and lumbar, all the way up to the neck and the base of the skull.

Breathing is the catalyst activating synergy to synchronize movement. Perform slowly to produce a well-prepared, strong, coordinated foundation that can handle increases of force, speed and intensity for progression. It all starts with breathing. Breathing and movement are about improving quality first, not quantity. We need the linkage and interactions between functions to produce optimal results as well as prevent pain and injury. Quantity will build from practicing quality. But quality will not build from just practicing quantity. Development is what you put in to reap benefit and reward. More is not better until you are functionally efficient and trained. Know this in strength training as well. Feeling tired from the breathing exercises is a sign that you need to rethink how you perform fitness, strength and conditioning programing even how you live life. You must consciously, consistently, competently practice to make it a habit. At any point go back and see if your breaths per minute lowered. If you get quick results, great! If not, trust that practice hacks away the barriers and years of dysfunction and inefficiency.

I always feel stronger after my breathing practice. It is the reason I get stronger in my second, third and fourth sets with strength and movement. The strength of the breath gets deeper and generates more power to produce more strength that is perceived by the neuromuscular and nervous systems. Strength progression relies on increased pressure, tension and stability. Breathing supersedes movement in developing strength. Therefore, strength increases in sets if you know how to use your breath in recovery and activity. You should be getting stronger in your sets, not weaker. This has much to do with the strength, stamina and endurance of your breathing to move loads in strength training.

The students I work with cannot believe how fast they start to move and how strong they become in one or two sessions. For example, a client I had in the past would press a weight 4 times the first set, 5 times the second set and 6 times the third set. Not bad for one session. But they all say the same thing—they realized they had been breathing in totally the wrong manner, which affected how they performed strength and cardiovascular exercise. They would say that the lack of endurance and strength in their breathing made them weaker and more tired. So, their strength decreased. Maintaining breathing pressure and tension over time causes strength to increase, not decrease.

Unfortunately, the mastery of breathing is pushed to the curb for the sake of strength training and quantity. Your regimen should be about how your movements strengthen your breath and your breath strengthens your movement. Think about exertion for movement and stabilization for a moment. To throw in judo, you need to breathe in as you are setting up the technique into the movement, to exhale at the throwing point. A rugby tackle or a defensive lineman in football's strongest point is on the peak of inhalation as he hisses for exhalation. For a hockey player's slap shot, he breathes in to wind up and exhales on the slap shot for power, likewise for a tennis swing or golf swing. What your sport or training is will define when to release the breath or when to breathe for power. Each way you see it there is transference of power from breathing to the core through movement. That's why you train breathing inside the movement patterns in the exercises and poses at the end of this book. The beautiful thing about breathing is, you can do it anytime, any day and anywhere. It works quickly. The hard part is making it habitual. **Your Breath Is Your Power.**

Chapter 6
GOT STABILITY??

"The physical world, including our bodies, is a response of the observer. We create our bodies as we create the experience of our world." – Deepak Chopra

THE CORE IS NOT JUST ABS

By this time you know what the core is and how it works from performing the breathing techniques. You now feel that breathing through your nose activates the diaphragm. You now understand that breathing is the primary mechanical component that is responsible for the respiratory, cardiovascular, musculoskeletal and nervous systems functional integration. Your core is the center of gravity that stabilizes the body in alignment as well as produces the power of movement.

On the physical level, if you draw a circle around the navel, the hips and the lower back, anything in this area directly affects and develops the core. Breathing, the abdominals, hips and spine comprise the core's functional pieces. The core is dependent on their function, position, stability and alignment to establish it's power source. The stronger the core, the more power you can produce, transfer, coordinate, synchronize and ramify through training, performance or daily movements. When you think about strength and power you should think about breathing and alignment to activate and power the core. Synchronization is the key.

Training the core requires you to train it in all movements, not in isolation like crunches'. The core is not isolated nor is it just muscular contractions, as society tends to think. People love doing crunches without having any knowledge about their ramifications. Crunches are detrimental, creating a strong abdomen but also wreaking havoc on the spine at rest, pulling it forward into poor posture. Exactly what crunches do, produce isolated strength that ramifies imbalance and weakness to other joints and muscles. There is no reciprocation. This imbalance renders the core ineffective because you are strengthening one muscle without the other. Muscles contract to stabilize joints in alignment for other muscles to stretch and move. What strengthens the core is everything working together not one specific thing. Over strengthening or weakness in one aspect of the core unconsciously sabotages alignment and balance. The core produces strength through balance and leverage that travels through the whole body, and is more advantageous than isolated muscular strength, such as crunches. Movements like crunches do not transfer into movement patterns no matter if you are standing up, playing rugby, soccer, running, wrestling or judo, etc. Muscular strength isolation produced from crunches, threatens to undermine movement performance and range of motion in movements like plank, pushup, overhead presses, dead lift, etc. where spinal alignment is essential to elicit the proper results. Training crunches for abdominal isolation develops strength that will work against itself, in sports performance, fitness classes and strength and conditioning training.

Without core stability in a squat, the spine moves forward; in a push-up the lower back sags; in a lunge the spine flexes forward, lifting the arm up causes the spine to lean to the side or hyperextend. When you run with the spine flexed, rounded forward, your joints and spine absorb more shear force, causing pain and strain because of poor core stability and possibly poor hip stability. Looking at the issues more closely through the functional microscope, breathing and the core tend to be the hidden, buried issues. People move and train unconsciously without alignment and a fully developed core.

It is important to train the core as the center of gravity and build strength there from different movements. The foundation for this type of training is to expose the core to many different positions. Training the core from different positions makes the core stronger at its primary functional position. Most people have it all wrong in strength training, only training the surface level of muscles not including breathing, alignment and stability in their approach. Training the core and the body in many different positions develops better performance and strength because of practicing leverage. As a result, it makes the center—the core—reactive, stronger, more coordinated, educated and perceptive, understanding movement.

One very important reason I wrote this book was for you to realize that movement was the third factor in performing a movement pattern, pose or exercise. When you create a movement like a lunge, pushup or squat, these movements are just movements that create tension for you to strength train your breathing, alignment and core. Most people see it in reverse, training muscles as the primary result. If you can't breathe functionally, no matter how much weight you can move, it won't work well in the world of practical movement. Without core stability in movement, you produce inefficient and compensated movement and transfer it into other exercises. Shifting the center of gravity has a more profound effect on movement than piling on weights for strength, especially for performance. Most people cannot master simplicity to function first in their own movement patterns using their own body weight before proceeding to add weights to their movements. Strength and power is like a wild horse, it is something you need to know how to harness, tame and move, not just develop.

Personally, I've experienced the importance of the core—from all the years of strength training, physical conditioning, playing soccer for sixteen years, rugby for seventeen years, and from all the years of wrestling and judo. Remember, that breathing and the core are crucial for endurance and stamina in a sixty-minute training session, a ninety-minute game, through your day and daily tasks. In rugby, you need the power of the core to sustain being tackled, tackling, holding up your opponent and to drive a maul, meaning driving an opponent off the ball. If you not familiar with the game of rugby, watch a game for a few minutes and you will begin to understand the importance of breathing and the core. In wrestling and judo the core gives you the necessary power you need through the arms and legs as leverage.

Without breathing, the core will not be coordinated and you will not develop reactions and reflexes for speed and transitions properly. You can move the biggest muscle guy with leverage and core power in rugby, judo or any sport. The stronger the core the more leverage you can produce. The key to leverage is the fulcrum. By increasing the strength of breathing and the core, the fulcrum, the levers get stronger to move. If the fulcrum gets stronger you can increase your strength training in short order. Learning to access the core will make the vital difference when progressing and evolving movement.

JOINT STABILITY

Joint stability is important in preserving joint alignment to maintain a functional, optimal and efficient position. Joint alignment dictates, controls and coordinates range of motion, muscle flexibility and mobility. By contracting muscles, you stabilize a joint's alignment, for example, the glutes and the hip joints. The glutes' strength and contraction keeps the hip joints in a stable aligned and balanced position. It prevents the hip flexor from developing too much tension, pulling the hips forward into a tilt decreasing range of motion and destabilizing the lumbar. Maintaining the hip alignment allows the opposing muscles, like the quads, to have optimal flexibility and range of motion and to contract for other muscles like the hamstrings to stretch properly. With joints like the knee and ankle, they will move more efficiently and effectively from an aligned joint position. A stable, aligned joint produces the best mechanical advantages for range of motion, joint mobility and flexibility.

Joint compensation and misalignment, on the other hand, is an unconscious process. Sitting too much, developing poor posture and breathing through your mouth are just a few examples of how the body unconsciously moves into misalignment and loses stability. When this shift happens, we are not mindful or aware of it because we don't feel it happen.

Joint stability is one of the most important factors in functional movement. It allows motion to transfer. Joint stability is needed to move and direct energy joint to joint. Each step you take to walk, run, jump, lunge, squat, push or pull is based on the stability platform. In a squat, if you round your spine or lean it too far forward, your core is not stabilizing. Poor core stabilization affects the ankles and knees losing all the stability that the core and spine transfers from an erect position. Try it. Lunge with just a little bit of range of motion. You don't need much to feel this example. First, use a rounded spine and lunge three times (photo 1). Now, pull your shoulders back or you can slightly hyperextend your spine (photo 2). Create core and spine stability the best you can and lunge three times. You should have felt a huge difference in transference of stability to the foot, ankle, knees and hips in the motion by just straightening your spine and pulling the shoulders back. You need stability and alignment to transfer forces properly through the body to create strength for the whole body, not isolated strength.

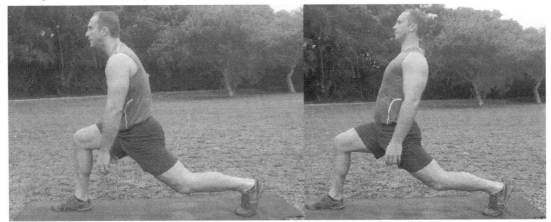

In photo one, the result is a lunge that moves but really does nothing for your body to strengthen breathing, the musculoskeletal, nervous and neuromuscular systems. What's more, in a shoulder press the lat and scapula muscles contract to stabilize the shoulder joint to press the weight and straighten your arm over your head. The lat contraction is absolutely necessary to stabilize and ground the shoulder joint for the arm to produce range of motion. If your spine is rounded forward, shoulder mobility is compensated and the joint has less range to produce motion because of misalignment of the spine, as you experienced in a previous chapter and can see in photo one above. As you keep loading the shoulder mobility without stability and alignment of the spine, pain ensues, impingement develops and injury is lurking. Your movement is ineffective. Consequently, you begin to transfer ineffectiveness to other movements, developing pain and the beginning of bad movement habits. You start to function differently for many movement patterns, poses or positions.

In my training, I focus on stability and alignment, and to move that stability and alignment into ranges of motion. I don't try to justify range of motion without the functional foundation. I use my joints to move and let the muscles respond by contracting to stabilize the joints' position to allow range of motion and flexibility to be optimal. I don't focus on flexibility programing. It happens through my strength and movement training. Flexibility is the result. For example, performing a body weight dip, I breathe in stabilizing the abdominals, contracting the lats and the back muscles and stabilize the scapulas. I contract the quads and glutes as well. This allows me to move into a deep range of motion with a straight spine. The same occurs with a push up. Breathing in to contract the abdominals and lats on the descent to the floor stabilizes the shoulder joint maintaining alignment that allows more range of motion to stretch the chest. As you ascend in the dip and pushup, keeping the lats contracted maintains scapula and shoulder joint stability and balances strength development between the chest and the back.

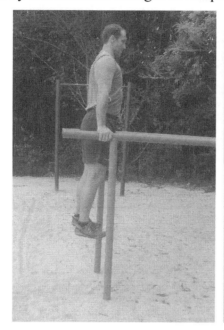 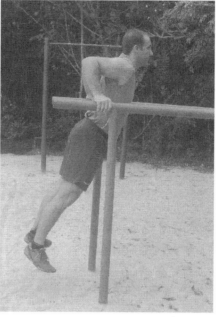

As my muscles stretch, it's not just a passive stretch it is a loaded controlled stretch through movement that augments strength. Similar to a cable holding up the span of a bridge, it is being stretched but maintaining its tension, power, strength and alignment without being overstretched to maintain the forces applied. The more you stabilize a joint in a movement, pose or exercise, the more control and strength you have to move into range of motion effectively. All this teaches your body and joints how to maintain alignment and produces the linkage, leverage and synergy to move and strengthen the whole body. The nasal diaphragmatic breathing initiates this whole process. Don't think about speed right now. Speed comes when you have control of the movement and all the functional integrations (stability, mobility, contraction and flexibility) that produce range of motion working together. Society misses this valuable piece of strength development by focusing on strengthening specific muscles, speed and how much weight they can move with a poor functioning body rather than strengthening the functional aspects for strength development and progression.

I see many people performing chest dips rounding the spine forward like photo 1 and 2 on the following page. They are strengthening misalignment and losing the development of the linkage in muscular strength. Just because you can produce more range of motion by compensating the spine to round forward, does not mean it is productive, much like the lunge you just performed. It does not have much development in strength but you can move forward more. People compensate joint stability for range of motion. Without the stability platform, you create force and imbalanced strength.

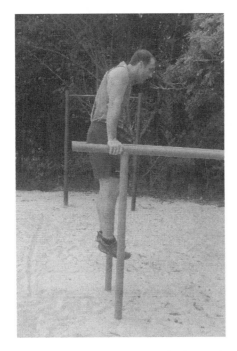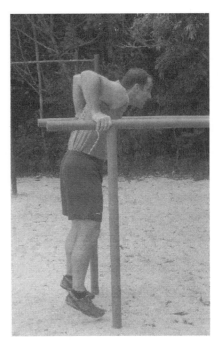

Stability creates the foundation, the structure, for movement to function. The foundation's stability is going to be a critical factor to support the forces imposed on the body. In the standing position, all the joints promote stability. The joints should all be in alignment in a standing position, that is, they should all line up in a straight line from ear to shoulder, shoulder to elbow, elbow to hip, hip to knee, and knee to ankle. If you lack alignment in the standing position, how does that transfer into movement? Your alignment is what moves you. Next is the Standing Postural Blueprint. This will help you understand your alignment better.

STANDING POSTURAL BLUEPRINT

Using the Standing Postural Blueprint, draw an imaginary straight line from your ear down to the outside of your ankle. Your ear should line up with the ankle joint to create a line of stability. Anything outside this line of stability develops shear force, placing excessive unnecessary strain on the structure. Shear force occurs when alignment is not parallel with the line of gravity.

According to the *Merriam-Webster Dictionary*, shear force is: "1. something resembling a pair of shears, 2. an action or stress resulting from applied forces that causes two contiguous parts of a body to slide relatively to each other in a direction parallel to their plane of contact." When joints are not stacked properly in alignment, gravity causes a shear force on joints in misalignment and poor posture. Alignment is straight and gravity lines are straight. As you move away from alignment the joints become vulnerable to the shear forces of gravity. When the cervical spines move forward like in the photo above in the dip and on the next page, when the ear does not line up with the

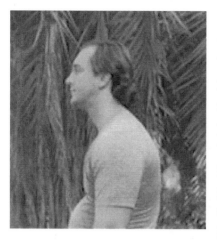

shoulder, they have lost their alignment. The interaction in working together with the rest of the spine and the body is lost. They now work separately to maintain misalignment resulting in a loss of flexibility, stability needed for range of motion and joint mobility. At this point, the muscles are contracted and stiff, especially in the back of the neck, to support misalignment's poor position, being affected by shear force. This position produces the "stabilizing factor" for the joint that is not aligned or balanced and therefore produces strain and has limitations to movement. Now their primary job is basically just to hold on because of gravity's pull. The more the cervical spines or any joints maintain poor position, the further the joints start to fall away from the body, the more it increases pounds of pressure from a rested standing or sitting position becoming strained, training the neuromuscular system to stabilize and lock in on that poor position. So, when the cervical spines move forward, it loses its ability to rotate side-to-side, look up and back because it is locked into flexion. Each time the cervical spines move, the mobility increases the pressure and tension on the joint that cannot be dispersed or transferred through the motion, especially in runners or anyone performing sports, exercise or fitness. As you can see, when the joints are absorbing tension and unable to transfer the signal to the next joint, movement and an increase in force makes the issue worse. Now imagine trying to progress strength training, fitness, yoga or any training program with the cervical spines or any joint misaligned this way. Being unconscious to this process is why pain and strain happen and how injury and disorders occur through time.

The Standing Postural Blueprint is a simple, effective way to look at the efficiency and effectiveness of joint alignment and the spine's posture. Joint alignment is an indicator and predictor of movement and is a good prevention tool for awareness before you move. Observe the side profile of your body, the back and the front. The easiest way to do this is to take a full-length photo of your body to get an accurate view. Use the timer on your camera or have someone take the picture for you. You can use video as well. Just start recording and stand in the frame sideways, back and front. Hold each standing position for about 10 seconds. Do what's natural to stand up straight. Do not exaggerate. See what your natural tendency is and what needs to be functional. See how your joints line up and how your feet are pointed. If you pose with good posture, you will miss the point of this technique.

Right away, you can see possible misalignments and asymmetries in alignment that will affect movement patterns, function and range of motion.

From the side, look at how:

- the ear is in line with the shoulder joint.
- the shoulder joint is in line with the elbow joint.
- the elbow joint is in line with the hip joint.
- the hip joint is in line with the knee joint.
- the knee joint is in line with the ankle joint.

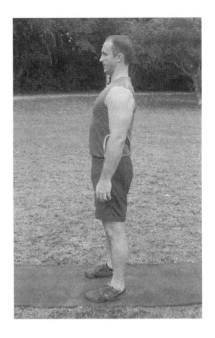

From the back and front:

- see if the shoulders have symmetry and balance.
- see if one knee is bent forward more than the other.
- see if you stand on one leg or sway the hips to one side.
- see if the hips have symmetry and balance.

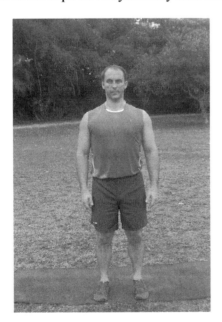 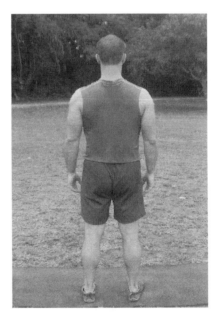

(When you look at the hips, look at the hipbones in the lower back.)
(When you look at the shoulders, look at the scapulas and the top tip of the shoulders.)

Looking at how the joints line up is best illustrated in the Standing Postural Blueprint. It shows where tension is imbalanced in muscles affecting the joints alignment. The hips, lumbar, thoracic and cervical spine, need to create alignment for effective whole body stabilization. The Standing Postural Blueprint shows if your head is too far forward, if your shoulders are slouching forward and if your hips are imbalanced. You will see where the joints line up and if there are possible stabilization issues from the start. Proprioception forms from the interaction with gravity pulling on our body's position and our responses to it.

If tension pulls forward, back or is stronger on one side, it produces imbalance. The hips will not be balanced and will have direct impact on how the spine and shoulders functions.

A LITTLE NOTE ABOUT BALANCED TENSION

Balance is the key for tension to be efficient and effective. When tension is balanced it maintains alignment, to hold up the structure of the body efficiently. When tension is not functioning well and is imbalanced, it will strain energy, muscles, joints and bones of the body. Excess is created on one side and weakness and deficiency on the other. This imbalance is what produces strain, pain and vulnerability to injury, where as alignment keeps it symmetrical and functional for optimal mobility. As you load forces on alignment, you produce strength balances. In misalignment, you can't move through a full range of motion to stretch and contract muscles in reciprocation of the movement. Loading forces on misalignments produce strength imbalances, creating strength on one side and weakness on the other because of the inability for certain muscles to contract optimally. For example, when lunging having tight hip flexors and weak glutes. You strengthen the muscular imbalances maintaining misalignment. In an athletic world this decreases performance limiting the athletes movement capability and potential. **Tension is efficient and effective when it is balanced working with the whole body rather than individual muscles producing strength imbalances decreasing motion.**

By performing the Plank Compressive Suit, you will feel how producing tension and joint stability strengthens and restores alignment, the center of gravity and how affecting one joint sets off the chain reaction and synergy for all, connecting tension through the joints and muscles of the body. Performing the Plank Compression Suit will help you understand how to fire the signals synergistically. Firing the Signals (FIS) will show you how muscular contraction is the trigger to a ripple effect for other muscles to reciprocate contraction as well as facilitate flexibility. For example, contracting the glutes automatically transfers tension and stability to the hips, abdominals, the lumbar, the back extensors of the spine and through to the arms and legs. It allows the hip flexor to be flexible. The next chapter will explain more about this topic. For now, let's try it.

PLANK COMPRESSION SUIT

When in misalignment or maintaining joint compensations, the body triggers ineffective joint-to-joint communication that does not transfer, reciprocate or act as a catalyst very well. Alignment is like a chain link that connects all the joints to work together. Performing a plank compressive suit squeezes all the muscles to hold an aligned plank position similar to that of an aligned standing position. In a plank, each joint is pulled down to the ground by gravity. You respond by contracting muscles to produce stronger and better joint alignment to develop and strengthen stability for the joints. Each joint is linked to the next joint through muscle tension; transferring the compressive tension forces through the musculoskeletal system of the whole body, joint to joint. As all the joints and muscles become involved and integrated, they interact, linking the whole body physically. Think of movement as a program and the structure of the body as the hardware. The respiratory, neuromuscular, musculoskeletal and nervous systems are the software. They all need to function together to run movement programs effectively like a computer.

Get into a plank position. Perform one at a time to feel the progression.

- Squeeze your glutes hard and notice how the abdominal stability reciprocates and counteracts. Notice how you feel the lumbar and back extensors of the spine. Feel the transference of stability by just squeezing the glutes. Feel the lats tighten as well through to your hands.
- Now, squeeze the quads with the glutes. Feel more tension in the kinetic linkage. This is tension strength activating the chain.
- Now, breathe into the abdominals with the bracing breath to create core stability with the contraction of the glutes, quads and abdominals. Keep it all tight and hold the plank for 5 to 10 seconds. Feel it through your hands and feet. As you contract muscles, you are increasing pounds of pressure, applying forces to the body.
- Now, add the lats by contracting the triceps. You should see the crease, the bend of the elbow face forward. Contract it all together. This is a plank.

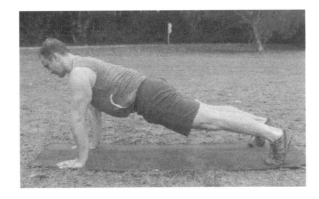

- **Optional.** If you can do a push-up with everything tight and compressed. Breathe in through the nose as you lower down to the floor, tightening and tensing the muscles. Breathe out, hiss, pushing up through the abdominal tension.
- **Optional.** Lean forward slowly over the wrists. This will improve the strength of the wrists, shoulders and lat.
- Train the plank using breathing repetitions. Breathe in, for example, for 5 seconds and exhale hiss for 3 to 5 seconds. Focus on contracting muscles on the inhalation harder and maintain the muscular contractions on the exhalation.

I wanted you to feel your core when performing the plank using FIS. When contracting the glutes you feel the abdominals and lumbar area react. And as you contracted the quads and incorporated inhalation with the glutes contraction, you felt the core area react stronger through connectivity. When you tense the glutes, quads and abdominals, you feel your hands' pressure on the floor. When you push up, you use the contraction of the muscles to stimulate the neuromuscular and nervous systems and stabilize to create leverage. Strengthening and applying tension to alignment increases the amplitude of the nervous system helping you do a push-up or any motion stronger using fulcrums and leverage because of using the joints and muscles and the integration of all the systems. I use this plank compression suit to help clients develop the strength to do a push-up that works very quickly. It also helps to understand, strengthen and restore alignment. This is what you want to feel in training and in performing movements. That's why I use slow movements first to develop strength and stamina activating the power in the nervous system to produce a natural effortless path for range of motion. I want you to understand how there is more to strength and movement than just moving. It is movement reciprocation, firing the signals (FIS), and the integration of the mind-body neuromuscular programing that will restore alignment to release the limitations and restrictions.

Training alignment and stability slowly is more effective in the beginning because stability has to coordinate into the timing and transference through the joints. You have to train the brain to process and develop what you are doing step by step to interact with movement. This creates a pathway of efficiency that improves the speed at which the brain can fire signals for muscles to move. The brain will record this and make a file as you practice consistently to keep the pathway active. This is identical to writing commands to run software. Once the brain can coordinate function, it can then synchronize movement, speed or intensity can be added. Like in a push-up, if your lower back keeps arching toward the floor (not the whole spine), you compromise core stability. If you train slowly by concentrating on breathing for core stability and contracting the glutes, you will have better support for the lower back to stabilize and transfer energy through the thoracic spine to produce stronger shoulder mobility and range of motion.

However, if you try to add speed without being functional, the timing, balance, synchronization of joints is not there; in contrast, this is what speed needs to function, a trained pathway. Be concerned with the quality of reps not how many or fast in the beginning. Doing a few good ones or learning the proper technique and approach for progression will develop more strength than doing eight or ten sloppy ones. When you train slowly the brain tames the urge for quantity because it is focused on quality. Only when coordination takes effect can you can add more speed or pace because you have cleared limitations in range of motion's pathway. If the timing is off in movement, it loses joint transference, communication and movement reciprocation. This is why movement reciprocation of joint stability and mobility, muscular contraction and flexibility is so important, as you will learn next.

If done too fast, muscles and joints don't know how to respond, especially in the beginning of a movement or training program. There is no trained neuromuscular, neurological pathway of development for movement. So, the brain does the best it can with what is available to move, for example, misalignment and asymmetry. Slowing movement down shows you what's weak, limited and dysfunctional. Speed, however, will work to further a dysfunctional state, unless you are functional for speed. The unconscious mind is smarter than you consciously. It makes changes and adjustments without you even knowing.

Chapter 7
Movement Reciprocation
"A man paints with his brains, not with his hands." –
Michelangelo

MOVEMENT RECIPROCATION, Firing the Signals (FIS)

Reciprocation is the act of exchange to create balance in an environment or a relationship. Movement reciprocation works on many levels. The brain sends a signal to contract or relax a muscle, opening the window of flexibility known as reciprocation. This is also called the agonist and antagonist theory. I call it FIS, Firing the Signals. The glutes contract and the hip flexors stretch; the biceps contract and triceps stretch; the triceps contract and the biceps stretch; and the quadriceps contract and the hamstrings stretch. Firing The Signals (FIS) develops the foundation of joint alignment and stability, balancing tension similar to the Plank Compression Suit. First, the contraction of muscles stabilizes joints to restore and maintain alignment. After you have alignment, you preserve alignment in motion by contracting muscles to reciprocate stretching for flexibility, range of motion and mobility. This is one way you gain back the resiliency of your youthful flexibility, to become stronger, move well and reverse pain. It is how you make yourself flexible and stronger when you thought you could not be. It just depends on how you move, what you are practicing and what you are doing in your life or work that is creating inflexibility, pain or strain. FIS will help you tune into timing and synchronicity for proper movement and strength production.

FIS is good to apply to asymmetry, misalignment and movement compensation that is inhibiting a movement pattern or range of motion. It will improve a joints position and angle to produce a greater range of motion properly. **The whole body's potential to move well depends on all the joints being aligned, and being able to stabilize that alignment to move.** The body is dependent on joint stability to create mobility through joint-by-joint communication. For example, performing a lunge, if the hip flexors are tight, they are inefficient and not very effective. Alignment starts at the center, the hips. The glutes strength prevents the hips from tilting, preventing the hip flexor from developing contractile tension that will render the hips to be ineffective to move well. As the hips lose alignment and balance, a series of compensations begin to develop. The dysfunction and compensations ramify through the whole body. The weakness of the glutes cannot contract to maintain alignment. The hip flexor and inner thigh create tension because of the lack of strength in the glutes, holding the hips in an ineffective misaligned position against gravity. To correct this issue you can simply strengthen the glutes, contracting them to stabilize the hips to reverse the series of compensations. It will push the hips back up into a balanced aligned position, returning the hip flexors' ability to stretch, be flexible and effective to move well and lunge. As you bring strength and balance back to the glutes, it produces better energy flow through movement and opens the functional path to train the spine and back muscles.

Something has to make up for the loss of alignment to maintain the balance. Restoring alignment is the best way to become flexible, improve mobility and avert pain and injury. If you keep stretching and stretching and you get little to no results or get results that keep returning to the same tension or see it getting worse, this is probably the reason why. There is no reciprocation. Be mindful to make all the mechanics synchronize to function, to stabilize the joints alignment and produce flexibility.

If you stretch muscles, you are trying to stretch a pattern that is not functional because:
- the joint is in misalignment or is in a poor mechanical position with limited range of motion.
- the muscle is tight, supporting the misalignment, losing its flexibility.
- the system is compensated how to move because of joint misalignment.
- muscular contraction is too weak to produce range of motion.

The inflexibility will not release until the joint is stable and aligned or the muscles are able to fully contract for muscle to produce optimal flexibility. You need to apply the following formula: *alignment + joint stability (muscle contraction) + muscle flexibility = range of motion.* If you apply this formula, you will start to gain inches of flexibility that will begin to train the brain to start creating more range of motion. It is how you increase the circuit's system power.

Without alignment:
- joints lose stability and muscles create tension and lose their natural flexibility to support the joint misalignment against gravity.
- you lose range of motion.
- misalignment increases risk to pain and injury in movement.
- all the systems compensate to stabilize misalignment.

Flexibility needs three things to be optimal to perform.
- Joint alignment.
- Muscles to contract to produce joint stability to maintain joint alignment.
- Muscular contraction to produce muscular flexibility.

Try this lunge exercise as an example of FIS, movement reciprocation, to understand it power.

- Place one knee on the floor. Place the other foot out in front and assume a lunge position. Squeeze the glute on the knee side that is on the floor **then stretch** the hip flexor second (most people only stretch a muscle).

- As you stretch the hip flexor, don't release the glute. Only go as far as the contraction will allow you, don't force the stretch. You will really feel the stretch with the glute contraction. The contraction helps create leverage and maintain alignment. If you force you will only cause the system to create inhibition. (If you stretch too hard too fast the muscle will constrict, closing the window of flexibility.) Motion will be limited.

- Once you find that point where the stretch stops, hold the contraction for 5 seconds and release. Return to the top of the lunge starting position and relax for about 10 seconds. Perform again, contract the glute and then stretch, holding the contraction for 5 seconds at the barrier, release and relax for 10 seconds. Perform a total of 3 times with 10 seconds' rest in between. The rest in between allows the proprioception system to scan and make adjustments for balance, alignment, stability and strength immediately. It writes a program that fast!

What you should have felt is: the glutes contracting harder, stabilizing the hip and moving deeper into the stretch, controlling the movement of the hip for the hip flexor stretch. You should have felt the lunge get deeper and deeper in each set. This preparation is so often missed in fitness and strength training as well as rehab and prevention. Try to feel the contraction and the stretch. If you feel you cannot contract muscle and stabilize the joint, feel if the opposition has tension blocking your movement. That's why you contract and stabilize first then stretch second. **Don't worry about how far you can stretch. Use the system and progression will happen.** If cramping occurs, it is a sign muscle fibers are weak. This usually happens in smaller stabilizing muscles, like the gluteus medius on the side of the hip. (When you are lying on your side and you lift your leg into the air, you will feel the gluteus medius muscles on the side of the hip. If they cramp, they are weak. Common for many people and a reason for knee and lower back pain.) Cramping should send a signal that the muscle is not really doing its job to stabilize the joint. Without stabilizers, larger primary muscles destabilize and collapse alignment making the foundation weaker and weaker, much like building a building without support beams to support the structure. Stabilizing muscles contract to secure the joint in alignment for range of motion to happen or to move extremities or other joints for mobility. By contracting certain muscles, you create stability, flexibility and range of motion using reciprocation. This produces the mechanical advantages to be effective for mobility and movement. Affecting one joint or muscle affects all of them for good and for bad. *Stretching tight muscles in misalignment only stretches tension. Stretching will, therefore, not fix the cause of tension and inflexibility.* The table below provides information about how movement reciprocation works. Mobility and flexibility responds to the position of joint alignment and posture.

Table 2 is based on a standing position for stability and mobility. This chart is based on single joint reciprocation to understand whole body movements.

Joint	Muscular Contraction	Muscular Flexibility
Calf Raise **Ankle** Toe Point	Calf Shin Muscles	Shin Muscles Calf
Leg Extension **Knee** Leg Curl	Quads Hamstring	Hamstring Quads
Lunge **Hip** Standing Knee Lift	Glutes Hip Flexor	Hip Flexor Glutes
Abduction **Hip** Adduction	Gluteus Medius Adductor (Inner Thigh)	Adductor (Inner Thigh) Gluteus Medius
Internal Hip/Foot Rotation **Hip** External Hip/Foot Rotation	Internal Rotators External Rotators	External Rotators Internal Rotators
Push Up **Shoulder** Back Row (Pull)	Chest Lats (Back Muscles)	Lats (Back Muscles) Chest
Internal Rotation **Shoulder** External Rotation	Internal Rotators External Rotators	External Rotators Internal Rotators
Bicep Curl **Shoulder and Elbow** Arm Extension	Biceps Triceps	Triceps Biceps
Wrist Curl **Wrist** Reverse Wrist Curl	Forearm Flexors Forearm Extensors	Forearm Extensors Forearm Flexors

Wherever you see or feel more tension, work on the opposite muscles to contract to restore strength balance to the joint. There are many more muscle movement reciprocations in the body. I wanted to point out the basic ones first for you to understand this concept. In the movement section you will perform exercises using muscle reciprocation and FIS.

Ankle Joint: CALF RAISE

When the calf or soleus gets too tight it pulls the foot down, keeping the ankle joint open; weakening the front of the ankle joint exposing it to forces through movement that it cannot stabilize to move. Calf raises contract and shorten the calf muscles, disrupting the balance of the ankle joint and shin muscle. It shifts the weight of the body to an anterior loaded position (shifting the weight forward) in the foot, reducing the foot's surface area on the ground. When the feet are flat on the floor with tight calves, other joints move from their alignment to compensate for this imbalanced tension.

Ankle Joint: TOE POINT

It is good to practice this movement to balance the ankle joint. It helps strengthen and contract the shin muscles, on the opposite side of the calves, pulling the toes toward the knee. Usually the calf muscles overpower the shin muscles. It gives strength and balance to the ankle joint; balancing the calf tension. The tibialis anterior, the shin, needs strength to stabilize movements, like a squat, lunge or in running. The ankle joint being able to close strengthens the shin muscle and transfers energy to the knee properly.

Knee Joint: LEG EXTENSION

The hamstrings' inflexibility creates a loss of the quadriceps' contraction and strength to extend the leg. The quadriceps' contraction stabilizes the knee in extension and transfers energy to the hip, extending the leg below the knee.

Knee Joint: LEG CURL

The hamstrings' contraction facilitates the stretch of the quadriceps. The quadriceps' tension can limit the hamstrings' curl.

Hip: LUNGE

When the hip flexor gets too tight it will tilt and pull the hips down and forward. When the hamstrings get too tight from sitting, it pulls the hips back, also tightening the hip flexors. Contracting the glutes will provide stability and balance for the pelvis. This enables the hip flexors and hamstrings to develop optimal flexibility and resiliency.

Hip: THE STANDING KNEE LIFT

When you lift your knee, the hip flexor contracts.

Hip: ADDUCTION and ABDUCTION

When the adductor (inner thigh) stretches the gluteus medius contracts on the side of the hip. When it is tight, the isolated tension of the adductor overpowers the gluteus medius to contract fully. The adductor tension stabilizes the hip isolating the tension between the inner leg, the hip and knee. Abduction is moving the leg back to the center.

Hip: INTERNAL ROTATION and EXTERNAL ROTATION

For the hip joints to internally rotate the internal rotators contract and the external rotators stretch. When the hip is externally rotated, the rotators contract and the internal rotators stretch. The internal and external hip rotator imbalance affects knee stability. It makes the foot pronate or invert when stepping or running. An example of external hip rotation is sitting crossing one leg over the other. Lie on the floor and rotate your feet inward, internal rotation, so the toes point at each other. Turn your feet out, external rotation, away from each other. You will feel the hip rotators by just the slightest movement of the feet. Looking at the toes, see if there is any motion difference and how it feels to rotate the hip joints, easily or with tension. The feet are controlled by hip rotation.

Shoulder: PUSH UP

In a push-up, on the way down the shoulders and lats contract for the chest muscles to stretch, like a pull. If the lats don't stabilize and contract, it pulls the shoulder forward out of alignment. On the push back up the chest contracts and the lats maintain their contraction.

Shoulder: BACK ROW (PULL)

When you pull, the scapulas stabilize and the lats contract. The chest stretches when the lats contract.

Shoulder Mobility: INTERNAL ROTATION and EXTERNAL ROTATION

The tension and imbalance of muscles and misalignment of the shoulder joint decreases shoulder mobility, restricting rotation internal or externally. Many people think they don't need to focus on internal and external rotation but that is exactly what the shoulder does, it rotates the joint internally and externally in all movements. Even in a shoulder press and lat pull down the shoulder joint rotates. If motion is stuck, then it applies force to the joint. The thoracic flexion, rounded spine, produces mechanical disadvantages for shoulder mobility and range of motion losing alignment and space. Lift your arm straight out to the side. Rotate your palm from down to palm up for external rotation and palm up to palm down to palm facing back for internal rotation. Feel what's happening.

Shoulder/Elbow: BICEP CURL and ARM EXTENSION

Bicep isolated strength can inhibit range of motion, hinging the elbow from straightening the arm. The bicep strength people concentrate on imbalances the strength of the triceps to contract. The biceps' strength tension imbalance pulls unconsciously forward on the shoulder joint. If the shoulder joints start to move forward you will lose scapular and lat stability, affecting the posture, rounding the spine.

Wrist: WRIST FLEXION and EXTENSION

Extensors or flexors can tighten and pull the wrist forward or back inhibiting wrist and hand mobility. Put your arm straight out in front of you with your palms down. Bend your hand and fingers down then up. Notice if there is any weakness or limitations in the movement.

Spine Reciprocation Chart

Joint	Muscular Contraction	Muscular Flexibility
Flexion (Looking Down) **Cervical**	Front Neck Muscles	Back Neck Muscles
Hyperextension (Looking Up)	Back Neck Muscles	Front Neck Muscles
Side Bend **Cervical**	Left Side Neck Muscles	Right Side Neck Muscles
Side Bend	Right Side Neck Muscles	Left Side Neck Muscles
Rotation **Cervical**	Left Side Neck Muscles	Right Side Neck Muscles
Rotation	Right Side Neck Muscles	Left Side Neck Muscles
Flexion **Thoracic, Lumbar**	Abdominals	Spine Muscles
Hyperextension	Spine Muscles	Abdominals
Side Bend **Thoracic**	Left Oblique	Right Lat Muscles
Side Bend	Right Oblique	Left Oblique
Rotation **Thoracic**	Left Oblique	Right Shoulder
Rotation	Right Oblique	Left Shoulder

Cervical Flexion: LOOKING DOWN

The neck flexors on the front of the neck contract and pull the chin and head down, stretching the muscles on the back of the neck. If the cervical spine has poor alignment and the neck muscles on the front of the neck are tight, it will prevent you from looking up effectively. If you look down constantly, like texting on your phone or at a computer, then the muscles in front of the neck will tighten and restrict the motion to look up.

Cervical Hyperextension: LOOKING UP
The neck extensors on the back of neck contract and pull the head back looking up, stretching the muscles in the front of the neck. This usually happens when the spine rounds forward into flexion.

Cervical: SIDE BEND
The muscles on the side of the neck contract as the muscles on the other side stretch when the head tilts to the side. You can often feel many differences between the left and right side because of using cell phone or holding a bag on one side.

Cervical: ROTATION
The muscles on the side of the neck contract as the muscles on the other side stretch when the head rotates left and right. You can often feel many differences between the left and right side. Using your cell phone or holding a bag on one side creates imbalances in rotation.

Thoracic/ Lumbar: FLEXION
When the spine rounds forward the abdominals contract and spine stretches. Looking at the dynamics of abdominal crunches, they create contraction, stretching the spine, pulling it forward into flexion. The straight back sit-up keeps the spine aligned and the abdominals stabilized to transfer through movements like a dead lift, lunge, etc.

Thoracic/ Lumbar: HYPEREXTENSION
When you hyperextend the spine you contract the muscles in the glutes, back and spine, and the abdominals stretch.

Thoracic: SIDE BEND
When you bend to the side, like the left side, the left oblique contracts and the right lat and side stretches and vise versa.

Thoracic: ROTATION
When you rotate to the side, the left side, the right oblique contracts, the left lat contracts and the left chest muscles stretch and vise versa.

THE X RECIPROCATION MOVEMENT PATTERN
When we begin to move the whole body in stepping, running, walking or lunging, we transfer our alignment through an "X" movement pattern. Step, stabilize, transfer and

move. When you walk or run, as your left leg moves forward off the ground to step, the right leg and foot stabilize on the ground that transfers stability to the left side of the hip and lower back, to allow the foot to lift and step properly. When you move, stability (the contraction of muscle) maintains joint alignment as the platform for other joints to move and stabilize as well as be mobile to produce movements like running, lunging, throwing, etc. There is a constant exchange of stability and mobility between the right and left sides as you throw, walk, run or lunge. For example to throw, you step with your left leg to transfer power to throw with your right arm. As you walk or run, the hip needs to be stable, aligned and balanced in order for the muscles on the side of the hip, the gluteus medius, to function properly, to stabilize. This becomes essential for the gluteus medius to transfer energy to the lower back. Right gluteus medius will transfer stability to the left lower back and vice versa, the X (Dr. Vladimir Janda). The gluteus medius is also important in transferring and activating stability to the knees as well. If a joint is not stabilizing, then tension does not transfer to other joints through the joint system, the tension, the force produced, injures the joint.

The following exercise will start to prepare a path and activate the signals for the X movement pattern, helping you understand this more thoroughly. After the corrective, you will learn to put all these exercises together.

Standing Hip X (Lumbar)
- Stand with your feet shoulder width apart.
- Place your left index finger and middle finger on the muscles above the hipbones in the lower back on the left side.
- Place the index and middle finger on your right hand on the right gluteus medius.
- Place all your weight on the left leg and foot to start.
- Shift to the right foot and then begin shifting back and forth many times. You don't have to do it fast.
- As you shift on to the right foot, you will feel the right gluteus medius and the QL above the left lower lumbar hipbones contract.
- Switch you finger position vise versa on the right lower back and the left gluteus medius and repeat. Feel for the impulse of the left gluteus medius and the right QL lower lumbar above the hipbones contract.
- This is the process that occurs when walking or running with each step. Standing on both feet brings stability to the hip (X) (left and right side).

When you lean your weight to one side or on one foot or leg than the other side when standing, it creates misalignment. The hip misalignment, for example where the hips shift to the left side, standing on the left leg, moves the hips away from the midline causing the straight leg or weighted side to be shorter while on the other leg the knee bends to maintain balance. When the hips shift in this manner, the side you are shifting to makes the hip slightly higher on that side than the other producing asymmetry. Now when you run or train with this issue, strength imbalances build and create limitations in motion from right to left sides. It is possible if you have a short leg, the cause can be poor hip alignment.

The problems lie in the functional circuitry, how the signal is transmitting. I simply wanted you to see how the signals work. The problem is, the weakness of the glute medius muscles affect the transmission of the signal. The unstable pelvis can show what and why muscles are tight supporting misalignment destabilizing the hip. For example, weak glutes = hip tilt, tight hip flexor; weak gluteus medius = tight adductor (inner thigh) and tight QL (Quadartus Laborum). When one muscle is weak especially a stabilizer, another muscle constricts to maintain structural integrity because another muscles is not functioning properly, leading to training or moving improperly. You can see the inflexibility and immobility trail starting because these compensations will lead to more, especially when the body starts to move. Depending on what kind of movement web you weave through your life with work, training, sitting or standing, etc., dictates how the body will be molded.

Throwing a ball with your right hand, you need your left leg to step, stabilize and move through the upper body to throw with the right arm. Our power is usually isolated to one side when we throw or kick a ball, depending on whether we are right or left handed or footed. When you kick a ball with your right foot, you step with your left foot to stabilize the kick of the right leg and foot through the ball, stability and mobility interaction.

As you step from the standing position into a lunge or run etc., it begins a series of reciprocations: stability, mobility, stability, mobility through your body's alignment/misalignment. Joint alignment and stability needs to be transferable from standing through movement to produce power.

You need the timing and sequencing for the signals to fire, to embed the pattern for the brain. The brain feels what is happening. Developing function this way makes strength more efficient, effective and safer.

Force creates inhibition much like forcing flexibility onto tension through a stretch. If you work on reciprocation and slowly on tension you will get more flexibility simply.

Chapter 8
Restoring the Functional Blueprint: Alignment
Resetting the Signals to Breathe, Stabilize and Move
" Lack of activity destroys good condition of every human being. While movement with methodical physical exercise save it and preserves it." – Plato

The brain is always scanning for efficiency. The minute something becomes inefficient or out of balance, the brain reformulates to produce the best position or functional process to survive. Balance is always sought and accomplished to be functional in the body whether it is for energy, digestion, misalignment or alignment. The body has to make it happen, functional or dysfunctional.

In a clock are many parts, and each part has a certain function to move or hold something in place for an overall objective—to tell the time. If a joint is misaligned, the timing chain is compensated or out of alignment to achieve the overall objective: to move efficiently, effectively and safely. It is unable to provide the proper function to coordinate movement. The information is perceived joint-to-joint or from tension in a muscle and like a finely tuned machine, the brain is right on top to make the necessary adjustments for compensation. It is always in your best interests for the body to adjust and compensate to help you avert pain and injury. It is not in your best interests to go play soccer, rugby, do yoga, CrossFit, run, jump, perform strength or power training under this compensation. Without pain you keep training what is limited, restricted an unconscious. Training with poor posture does not improve posture. It strengthens poor posture's position. The strength produced increases tension that is not calibrated through alignment. The misalignments and compensations need to be corrected and trained to become functional again prior to any movement training or intensity.

BREATHE INTO STRETCH (BIS)

Your goal or sport determines what type of breathing pace or rhythm you will use. The Breathe, Stabilize, Move Function First Method uses nasal diaphragmatic breathing to develop and train your breathing to support alignment and stability to move with good habits. It is a superior way to breathe for sports, exercise or fitness. Inhalation produces tension, stimulating the nervous system that increases the power of muscular contractions. The exhalation is the release of the inhalations power to move. Just like a balloon, the more air that is in the balloon the more force is released when air is released. The less air in the balloon, less force is released. As you breathe into the core you will feel the core like the expanded balloon and muscles contract harder through the body. As you exhale when the air is released like the expanded balloon, you will feel the muscles release power through motion.

BIS is a good way to learn how to coordinate the timing of your breath into a movement. For example, when you squat or lunge, breathing into the core supports the contraction of muscles and stability as you move down into a squat or lunge. As you stand up out of your squat or lunge, the exhalation is releasing the power of the inhalation. Secondly, when you breathe in, you bring power to the core and spine to stabilize alignment as well as for muscular contractions that facilitate the stretch reflex for muscle flexibility. The quickness of your breathing depends on the activity being performed that you need to train. If you are not breathing and using the core, you will not feel this power.

Breathe Into Stretch	Firing the Signals
Deep breathing to strengthen muscular contractions.	Contracts muscles to produce and facilitate flexibility.
Maintains the core's power and hip and spine alignment through movement.	Contracts muscles to produce joint stability and maintain a joint's alignment.
Increases pressure and tension in the core for musculoskeletal and neuromuscular power. Increases contractile power.	Increases power in the nervous system and muscular contraction power.

BIS uses the slow bracing breath to specifically stabilize the core and spine for movement to occur (slow to produce feed forward). As you create range of motion or a stretch, you will fire the signals through the movement. As you produce movement you integrate all the functions and systems to synchronize (respiratory, musculoskeletal and neuromuscular) creating a pathway.

You are always in control of your breathing and stability through movement. If you lose control of breathing, you are lowering your potential. Maintaining core tension can be a challenge. During the exercises if you want to breathe out at the top, it's OK to reset the breath and start again. Always remember you need to produce a functional system first to progress the strength of its functions.

- Start where you are comfortable.
- Notice that you may need to breathe before you move. As this happens, the breath is getting deeper into the core and adapting to create energy conservation by taking deeper breaths corresponding to the movement pattern.
- As your nasal diaphragmatic breathing becomes deeper, your movement patterns will increase in range of motion and strength. Breathing becomes efficient for

movement to be more effective and coordinated.

- Remember, more breaths equal's more energy usage and leads to fatigue.

The stronger the pressure produced from the breath, the stronger the core tension and transference through movement. These techniques integrated with firing the signals will make you instantly stronger because you are using the respiratory system to tap into the musculoskeletal and neurological systems. That is why I say the mind is 95 percent of your power. The strength of the breath, the core and spine stability will determine the future of your power and the function of your movement. *Train the integrations as one for empowerment. Without training the nervous system, the musculoskeletal system will not have true power and guidance.*

APPLYING BIS AND FIS TOGETHER

When performing BIS and FIS, do all the movements and techniques slowly to develop coordination, synchronization, balance, symmetry and alignment, for all the signals to fire and work together. Once you have synchronization of BIS and FIS, train it consistently and repetitiously for resiliency. Once they all synchronize, you can add speed. Speed needs a pathway. Slow movements will create the pathways for speed. The brain learns from this process of moving slow, integrating all the functions as one, reproducing it again and again for the future of movement. Slow movement acts as a feedback control system to adapt, adjust and change as needed. The brain produces a file, like a computer system, to hold information based on how the movement functions. If you cannot perform an exercise or movement slow, it is not going to happen correctly when you do it fast. Speed is based on what is present in your body. You cannot develop alignment and function through fast movement. Fast movements are based on reactions and training from the joints' positions and muscles that are trained through alignment and slow movements first. Since strength, speed and power are built on top of a functional foundation, all the functions need to be reciprocating and working together.

The cerebellum may act as a feedback control system for slow movements and a feed forward controller for fast movements. (From University of Texas Health Science Center at Houston – http://neuroscience.uth.tmc.edu/s3/chapter05.html)

ORDER OF FUNCTIONAL ALIGNMENT: Correcting the Blueprint

Shifting stability from the center of the body to the left or right means making adjustments to maintain posture and structure. Fixing the hips and spine first corrects many joint deficiencies. Fix the structure, restore alignment and like dominos joints and muscles start to fall into place with proper function, stability and mobility in balance, shifting the proprioception and awareness to the correct position. As joints become more functional and aligned, you will feel energy, lightness, warm, stimulated, youthful and awakened. Your posture and joints will feel better, have more range of motion and movement will be easier. This is also why people feel youthful and energetic.

Following the order of functional alignment will show you the root causes for:
- any restriction in range of motion,
- joint instability,
- asymmetry,
- pain, strain or
- any strength imbalances that may falter under load, forces being applied.

This will prevent pain, strain or injury by catching the corrupted issue first. Issues are easily correctable. Once injury happens, you can't go back and you need rest and treatment. Prevention is lost.

Hips First

The hips are first to be restored in the order of functional alignment because they are the center that affects the whole chain of alignment and movement. It is the first functional piece to be restored to produce the platform for all other joints to fall into proper functional position. Adjusting one adjusts all. Many joints and muscles suffering from strain and pain start to get better as the primary functional efficiency returns to the hips. It will start to resolve any lumbar, thoracic, cervical, shoulder, knee or ankle issues. The adjustment of the hips affects the position of the spine. The position and alignment of the spine determines and dictates the alignment, function and range of motion for the neck, shoulders and arms mobility. That's why it is important to have alignment before any fitness, strength, training, sports performance program or for everyday life because you move from this alignment and stability daily. The first step in restoring stability and balance to the hips is strengthening the glutes' to produce alignment and symmetry. The glutes' strength produces optimal flexibility and range of motion for the muscles of the legs. But, most importantly in the process of strengthening the glutes' to produce hip alignment is that it instantly activates the abdominals and the pelvic floor muscles, realigning the stability of the lumbar spine. If the hips are tilted forward and the spine is hyperextended, the lumbar is compressed and too tight and therefore the abdominals and pelvic floor are not so active. If you lift your arm up from this position, you will feel compression in the lumbar, not stabilization from the abdominals in this position. If the hips are tiled back, the spine rounds forward into flexion, losing alignment where the abdominals and pelvic floor become too tight. These muscular restrictions hold the spine in flexion preventing the arm from lifting straight above your head. When joints are in misalignment, strength is out of balance producing an anchoring effect that limits mobility and restricts motion. Simply producing balance and alignment will release restrictions and limitations for energy efficiency and effective range of motion. Once you have efficient and effective alignment, you strengthen that alignment that transfers and increases the strength of motion.

Correcting the hips' alignment first helps adjust and correct the spine's alignment and position. The spine is dependent on the hips position. You can correct the spine first but only attain limited progression or the problem can return if the hips are the primary issue. These misalignments are the start of a compensated, dysfunctional path that will ramify through the system, training and moving each day. This example here will teach you how the hip imbalance and compensation affects the spine.

Stand up. Push your hips back, slightly rounding the lower back as in **photo 1.** (Don't force it. This example is to teach you about misalignment.) Now try to lift your knee. Change the position of your hips to be forward as in **photo 2** and lift your knee. It's a big difference! You don't feel pain, but you can see there are limitations and restrictions developed by misalignment compensating the height that you can lift your knee. Because the hips are the center of alignment, the imbalance 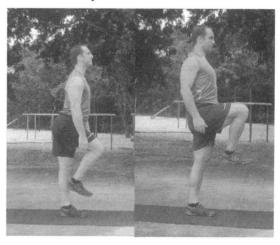 and misalignment sets off a chain reaction of other misalignments and dysfunctions, causing compensations to happen. When one joint adjusts they all adjust to produce a seemingly quasi alignment to stabilize against gravity. Another example to try is this. Move your hips forward and then back. Feel the whole spine naturally adjust its position from the movement of your hips. If your hips move back, the spine moves forward. If your hips move forward, the spine moves back. If you move the hips left, the spine moves right. If the hips move right, the spine moves left. The hips are like a gyroscope to move the spine. When the hips know the center, the spine will have stability. Think on the compensated level for a moment about how those adjustments above hold the spine incorrectly everyday or in fact how all the joints perform this process. If the hips are not aligned and stable in a movement like a squat, then other joints need to compensate to allow movement to happen.

Spine Is Second
Breathing has a profound effect on the spine's stability as well as the abdominals working in reciprocation and transference patterns with the spine. The abdominals help support the cervical, thoracic and lumbar spine and are just one piece of many that make

up the core. The abdominals are affected by pressure produced from nasal diaphragmatic breathing using the diaphragm. This process gets transferred to the spine to function and stabilize. For example, the abdominals (rectus abdominis) in the center from the top to bottom control flexion, stabilization and extension of the spine. Sit-ups pull the spine into flexion by contracting the abdominals and rounding the spine.

The obliques, on the sides of the abdominals, control the opposite shoulder (right oblique, left shoulder) in spinal rotation. If the spine is pulled into flexion (rounded spine), the rotation of the obliques or the side bend produces dysfunction. You are inadvertently training outside the line of alignment and stability for the spine. The spine is exposed to shear forces because of flexion. When performing rotation it adds intensity to the exposure of those shear forces. Although you are building strength, you are severely weakening alignment. As strength goes up with misalignment, functional movement becomes limited and inefficient rather than integrated.

The transverse abdominal is the compressor, the stabilizer that stabilizes through all spinal movements', flexion, extension, hyperextension and rotation. Nasal diaphragmatic breathing or the bracing breath integrates all the abdominal muscles to stabilize on a single breath. Try it. Breathe in deep through your nose and put your fingers on the different abdominal muscles and feel them tighten and react based just on your breathing. This cannot achieve this through mouth breathing. When mouth breathing and the abdominals are weak in stabilization, the core is disconnected.

Gravity will naturally and unconsciously pull any weakness forward, putting more stress on misalignment. When the spine rounds forward you create excessive forces at rest that cannot be transferred properly that remain imbalanced and excessive through movement.

STRETCHING THE SPINE

According to Dr. Stuart McGill, overstretching damages the spine muscles and ligaments. It may feel good but unrestrained stretching does damage in the long run. You may lose the stretch reflex, a protective mechanism. Furthermore, the spine is already overstretched in flexion, so there is little reason for more stretching; more stability and contraction is what is needed to make the spine erect and decrease the strain of gravitational forces. If you are unable to contract those muscles in the spine, then you should not be stretching those muscles. Most issues in the back and spine are due to muscles being taunt or overstretched already, hence, rounded spine. Your brain and body need to learn extension. You should not be performing any fitness programs without developing the hip/spine stability for alignment first because range of motion is based on this alignment. You can't stretch the spine if there is nothing supporting its' alignment and reciprocation to pull you back and balance you against gravity. Stretching the spine without alignment and core development will stretch open the spine vertebrae more than is necessary. By creating excessive flexion, you cause the proprioception system to alter and compensate function and efficiency. Proprioception will make adjustments based on the lack of stability and strength to find efficiency through compensation.

A more functional approach is to work on contracting the muscles to support and create your posture for extension of the spine. Contracted muscles of the back and spine pull you back to balance gravity pulling you forward. Without extension and posture of the spine, you lose the ability to coordinate movements. In the overstretching formula, flexion + flexion = more flexion. Behind the scenes, overstretching = imbalance + disharmony. Flexibility needs joint stability and alignment for optimal range of movement and stretch. McGill says stretching may feel good, but it's doing damage a little bit each time. It feels good because the proprioception system is trained in the art and mastery of joint compensation. Discomfort causes you to stretch because of the compensation and misalignment maintained over the years. The spine will feel more comfortable in its compensated position.

The problem is not truly with flexion. The problem is, not knowing how to control flexion to maintain alignment and stability, not having the strength to withstand gravity's pull forward. People start to stretch their spine without any functional information because of tension or pain. There is too much emphasis on stretching and rolling the spine. If the spine muscles can stretch, then they need to contract. It needs reciprocation as well and herein lies the problem. If your spine is not stable, stretching it will be detrimental. When the brain does not know how to move the body, it will move poorly through a conjured up compensated program unconscious to you. It is the reason why people get hurt in strength conditioning, yoga and stretch classes—they try to force a stretch or a movement without having proper stability and alignment from joints and muscles to contract, to direct movement forces. For example, in the downward dog yoga pose, with a flexed forward spine and no core development, the back extensors become strained. What's more, it's common for people to do a reverse plank, throwing their feet over their head, while lying on their back on the floor. You see people trying to stretch and force their legs over their head in an effort to stretch the spine. They simply don't have the function to accomplish this task nor will practicing this routine over and over help. Forced stretching produces inhibition in the stretch, flicking on inhibition signals to limit range of motion when too much tension cannot disperse or transfer. Again, it is done unconsciously because forcing a stretch instead of easing into it **slowly** with reciprocation calls for inhibition. The force and stretch are working against the brain's inhibitory responses. Meanwhile, you are consciously trying to create flexibility overriding the brain's commands. Force will not help your body become flexible nor will speed improve alignment The same goes for adding speed without preparation of movement. How can you add speed to the body in motion when it is sending inhibition signals and has limitations? We have the power to override the brain's commands of unconscious knowledge and we also have the power to tap into it.

It is OK to train flexion of the spine in movement patterns to contract and stretch muscles to maintain and retrain the spine's functional position. We use it to bend over to put on socks and shoes, etc. But some people are stuck in flexion and use it excessively and it progressively gets worse. And, some people are stuck in hyperextension. Again, the lack of aches, strains and pains make us think everything is ok. Training flexion is used as a means to restore balance, symmetry and alignment. It is NOT OK to use spinal flexion under loaded movements like a dead lift or a squat or to sit or stand in this position all day. The neutral spine position and the nasal diaphragmatic breathing pattern is used specifically to maintain alignment as well as prepare you to load movement to prevent shear loads from entering the spine and other joints.

Gravity mostly affects the thoracic spine, pulling you forward in what is called flexion.

After making the functional connection with your breathing, hips and spine, especially the thoracic in Level 1 and 2 routines, see what balanced out in your scapular stability, shoulder mobility and cervical movements. See if they feel better with less pain or if it takes less stress to move. Notice if your body feels lighter. Thoracic correction will automatically lead to improvements in the neck and shoulders to function and move balancing the musculoskeletal system. Restoring alignment and balance produces better energy. It works that fast and is that easy to correct alignment to start moving better.

PERFORMING THE CORRECTIVE MEASURES

- Focus on building the movement from the foundation of alignment, from in to out not out to in. This allows you to tap into the neuromuscular system.
- Feel the reciprocations. Don't just do mindless movement. That does nothing to connect your mind and body.
- Don't force. Use the functional system. For instance don't force a stretch and don't force a joint into position. Contract the muscles to produce alignment and flexibility.
- Work at establishing alignment and the correct signals for timing and synchronization of joints in movement. Train integration as one.
- Use rest in between sets for the brain and proprioceptive system to adjust and adapt to what was just performed. When the brain and body know what to do, rest time can be decreased.
- Produce consistency through the routine. What you do is what get's recorded by the brain.
- Perform regularly and often if not everyday to produce good habits.

Only move forward with progression when balance and alignment are achieved in the connectivity phase. If you move forward without balance you will not achieve optimal integration and linkage through the joints, maintaining compensation or asymmetrical strength. There are many times I need to work on connectivity from sitting too much some days, like when writing this book. When your body did the movement before it remembers how to do it again. You just get a little rusty.

NOTE: The previous exercise you do, creates a shift in the body. Correcting one joint affects other joints and muscles, and so on. It is the reason you restore alignment, strengthen the weakness and correct asymmetries first. Make the functions work inside the movement. Don't just move.

If you find that an exercise is easy, simply go to the movement encyclopedia and choose another one above it in the list. I have them ordered from easy to difficult so this way you can put your own program together following the Order of Correction.

HOW TO USE THE BREATHING CYCLE

The inhalation stabilizes the core and spine, contracts muscles to stabilize joints and loads the stretch. The exhalation releases the power through the mobility and movement. One breathing cycle is an inhalation and an exhalation.

In the first breathing cycle:
- Breathe in deep to stabilize the abdominals and bring power to muscles to contract as well as to stabilize joint position and alignment as you begin the movement. Once you reach the point where the motion stops in the movement hold the contraction and stretch for 3-5 seconds. You should be at the apex of the breath.
- Then from the held position (Don't move back to the start position. You will be in mid position.) exhale hiss maintaining or increasing the muscular contraction and stretch. There should be more movement in the range of motion. If not, feel for the ease of the position.

In the second breathing cycle:
- In the same mid position, new position after the exhale, breathe in again focusing on contracting and stretching those same muscles. Notice if the breath gets longer.
- Exhale again into the motion contracting and stretching those muscles maintaining alignment.

Perform this breathing technique for 3-5 breathing cycles in the movement. The first two cycles work at activating and integrating the circuitry. The next 2 to 3 cycles you start to feel the ease and see the range increase. If you have little to no motion, it's ok, keep working with repetitions.

You can also use the same breathing technique as above but instead, return to the starting position and rest 10 seconds after each repetition if you want. I am more concerned about the breathing cycles connecting to abdominal stability, muscular contractions and the stretch, to produce a neuromuscular pathway recognized by the brain for the musculoskeletal system and motion to develop properly. Breathing connects the nervous, neuromuscular, musculoskeletal and cardiovascular systems. You now see why breathing is the most important thing for movement, strength and power. If you don't practice it, it will not develop producing a compensated sub par system. Because breathing produces pressure and tension for the core, and the core is responsible for transferring power, it is essential to train breathing through movement. Breathing is the difference between becoming an athlete or a champion.

ALWAYS DO A PROPER WARM-UP FOR THE BODY BEFORE PERFORMING THE ORDER OF CORRECTION OR ANY TRAINING.

LEVEL 1-FOUNDATION

Hip and Spine Exercises – Producing the Foundation

Make the functions work inside the movement.

Perform:

- 3-5 breathing cycles in each position for 3-5 sets. (For example, if you do 3 breathing cycles, that's 1 rep.
- Perform each group first. In each group perform one exercise then the next. (For example perform the Lunge, Hip Bridge, Face Down Knee Lock Leg Scissor then the Lying Down Knee Lift as the first set and repeat for desired number of sets.
- Rest 10 seconds in between sets.
- Perform all the exercises applying BIS and FIS to produce the mechanical advantages for movement.
- Focus on contracting and stretching muscles with the breathing cycles.
- Apply 2 more reps and 3 more seconds to the weakness.

Group 1

Lunge Knee on the Floor- Page 115-116
Hip Bridge- Page 143
Face Down Knee Lock Leg Scissor- Page 148
Lying Down Knee Lift- Page 124

Group 2

Side Leg Raise- Page 125
Single Leg Frog- Page 137
Single Leg Hip Hinge- Page 130,131

Group 3

Seated Spinal Flexion/Hyperextension- Page 159
Seated Spinal One Arm Reach Side Bend- Page 160
Seated Spinal Rotation- Page 161

As you become proficient with each movement, you can add more mobility to the movement. Now that the hips have a balanced foundation for the spine, other joints and muscles will function properly. Many times the body regresses, like from sitting, and you can find issues that you may not have noticed disrupting alignment and movement. Level One will retrain the respiratory, musculoskeletal and nervous systems integration for joints and muscles to adopt alignment and produce good movement habits.

LEVEL 2-CONNECTIVITY

Add the abdominal exercises to improve connectivity to the hips and spine. Once you develop the foundation and the core is formed, you can add exercise and start your routine from the center.

- 3-5 breathing cycles in each position for 3-5 sets. (For example, if you do 3 breathing cycles, that's 1 rep.
- Perform each group first. In each group perform one exercise then the next. (For example perform the Lunge, Hip Bridge, Face Down Knee Lock Leg Scissor then the Lying Down Knee Lift as the first set and repeat for desired number of sets.
- Rest 10 seconds in between sets.
- Perform all the exercises applying BIS and FIS to produce the mechanical advantages for movement.
- Focus on contracting and stretching muscles with the breathing cycles.
- Apply 2 more reps and 3 more seconds to the weakness.

Group 1
Lunge Knee on Floor Side Bend/ Hyperextension- Page 117,118
Side Leg Raise Knee Bend Leg Extension Kick- Page 126
Frog- Page 139,140

Group 2
Single Leg Hip Bridge Knee Bend- Page 144
Face Down Knee Touch Leg Curl Lift Leg Extension- Page 149
Hip Hinge Close Stance Squats- Page 132

Group 3
Lying Down Knee Rolls- Page 175
Side Plank- Page 181,182
Straight Back Sit Up Knees Bent- Page 176

Group 4
Low Kneeling Spinal Flexion High Knee Hyperextension- Page 167
High Knee Spinal Rotation- Page 169
Plank- Page 189

- Slow and controlled in the beginning produces proficiency for speed and power.
- Move to the next exercise when you can do proficiently.
- Keep doing the exercises that still need proficiency. You may notice some exercises move forward and some remain the same.

LEVEL 3- INTEGRATION

In this level you will integrate shoulder and cervical mobility to hip and spine connectivity.

- 3-5 breathing cycles in each position for 3-5 sets. (For example, if you do 3 breathing cycles, that's 1 rep.
- Perform each group first. In each group perform one exercise then the next.
- Rest 10 seconds in between sets.
- Perform all the exercises applying BIS and FIS to produce the mechanical advantages for movement.
- Focus on contracting and stretching muscles with the breathing cycles.
- Apply 2 more reps and 3 more seconds to the weakness.

Group 1
Lunge Knee on Floor Hyperextension/ Flexion/ Rotation- Page 119,120,121
Side Leg Raise Knee Bend Leg Extension Leg Curl- Page 127
Face Down Knee Touch Leg Curl Lift Leg Extension Scissor- Page 150

Group 2
Single Leg Hip Bridge Knee Bend Lever- Page 145
Single Leg Frog Leg Extension- Page 138
Lying Down Knee Bend Leg Extension - Page 133

Group 3
Lying Down Knee Lift Alternating Leg Extensions Up- Page 177
Side Plank Leg Lift- Page 183
Alternate One Arm Plank Walk Up Overhead- Page 190

Group 4
Arm Bar Waist Wrap Cervical Rotation- Page 195
Upright Rows High Pull- Page 200
Cervical Lat Tension Flexion, Hyperextension, Side Bend, Rotation- Page 170,171

Keep mastering simplicity in each level so the advanced becomes simple and strength becomes advanced.

Chapter 9
Beyond Functional Efficiency: The Art of Progression
"When one has reached maturity in the art, one will have a formless form. It is like ice dissolving in water. When one has no form, one can be all forms; when one has no style, he can fit in with any style." – Bruce Lee

What you should have noticed by now is that you need breathing, alignment and stability to get optimal function, flexibility and efficiency for movement. When you have it, you can fit in with any style of training. The breathing techniques are designed to improve breathing and power to the core that works with life, fitness and sport. The breathing cycles train and develop the "energy reactor" on every breath. That's why you get more range of motion and become stronger instantly from using your breath. The muscles are like electrical wires that transfer energy to the joints that are like electrical boxes that direct the information to move; all connected to the core.

When you train BIS and FIS slowly, feel the contraction and lengthening of muscles. Don't just go through the motions to do it fast. Sloppy movement does nothing for proprioception. The power is using the functional circuitry, not just stretching or contracting to perform the pose. What happens inside the movement is what develops power and BIS and FIS will supercharge your strength training. It's the reason why my clients all got stronger in the 2nd and 3rd sets of their workout.

You don't need muscle failure and shallow fatiguing breath to get a good workout. Remember, your brain is recording what you do and builds a system around your functional performance. This is how it learns to be efficient, effective and progressive. Whatever is happening in your neurological world becomes your life and performance. If you sit with poor posture everyday, developing pain in the back, your body has to learn to transport that day to day and deal with it. If you are overtraining to the point of fatigue with sloppy posture, note that the brain produces and builds a system around that.

STRENGTHENING THE KINETIC LINKAGE

The key here is slow movement and strengthening the connection and integration of the respiratory, musculoskeletal and neuromuscular systems.

Level 4 – LINKAGE

Here you will combine two movements into one.

-3-5 sets for 5 reps, holding the contraction for 3 seconds.

-rest 10 seconds in between sets.

-perform all the exercises applying BIS and FIS to produce the mechanical advantages for movement.

-apply 2 more reps and 3 more seconds to the weakness.

Group 1

Lunge Knee Off Floor Knee Bend Leg Extensions- Page 122

Face Down Scorpion Leg Scissor- Page 152

Lying Down Knee Bend Leg Extension Hip Rotation Lateral Drop- Page 141

Group 2

Single Leg Hip Bridge Knee Bend Lever Leg Extension- Page 146

Lying Down Side Bend Leg Scissor Hip Rotation- Page 128

Hip Hinge Reach Back Y- Page 134,135

Group 3

Straight Back Sit Up Alternate Single Leg Lever- Page 178

Side Plank Leg Lift Arm Reach- Page 184

Plank Leg Lifts- Page 191

Group 4

Arm Bar Mid Back Lift Arm Extension Cervical Rotation- Page 196

T's- Page 201

Cervical Shrug Retraction Rotation- Page 173

LEVEL 5- SYNERGY

Don't add more exercises, add more motion to the exercise.

-3-5 sets for 5 reps, holding the contraction for 3 seconds.

-rest 10 seconds in between sets.

-perform all the exercises applying BIS and FIS to produce the mechanical advantages for movement.

-apply 2 more reps and 3 more seconds to the weakness.

Group 1
Synergy Lunge- Page 123

Face Down Scorpion Leg Scissor Side Bend- Page 153

Face Down Windmill- Page 154

Group 2
Single Leg Hip Bridge Knee Bend Lever Leg Extension Lateral Drop- Page 147

Hip Hinge Lat Rotation- Page 136

Alternating Lateral Squat- Page 142

Group 3
Straight Back Sit Up Single Leg Lever Leg Extension Up- Page 179

Side Plank Leg Lift Arm Reach Elbow Knee Touch- Page 185,186

Plank Opposite Arm and Leg Lift- Page 192

Group 4
Arm Bar Lift Extension Side Rotation- Page 197

Chicken Wings Up and Down- Page 203

Kneeling on Hands Cervical Rotation- Page 174

THE SITTERS ROUTINE

It can be close quarters in the office. It is probably difficult moving around on the floor especially with your boss near by. This routine is designed to help you avoid poor posture, misalignment and many other issues that affect your body throughout the day from constant sitting. Make it a habit to stand up 5-10 minutes every hour to perform this routine. You have to be mindful and practice if you want to change. Perform 3 to 5 sets for 5 repetitions.

Group 1
Lunge Knee on Floor- Page 115, 116
Seated Single Leg Extension Hip Rotation- Page 157 or 158
Single Leg Hip Hinge (Foot Assisted or Chair Assisted)-Page 130, 131

Group 2
Seated Spinal Flexion /Hyperextension- Page 159
Seated or Standing One Arm Reach Side Bend – Page 160 or 164
Seated Lat Rotations- Page 161

Group 3
Arm Bar Waist Wrap Cervical Rotation- Page 195
T's- Page 201
Cervical Spine Lat Tension Flexion /Hyperextension/ Side Bend Rotation- Page 170, 171

Group 4
Floor Desk Stretch- Page 205
Fist To Finger Flexion Extension- Page 207
Figure 8's- Page 204

I wanted to offer you a few different routines to build the structural functional integrity to move and for you to see your own progression. Preparation is prevention and prevention is strength. Everybody needs preparation for strength training, physical training and daily activities, to prevent moving like a "tin man". From the NFL and NHL players to the corporate office worker to the elderly population, everyone needs to be functional first. Who you are, does not matter. The functional level provides the opportunity to prevent pain, strain, injury diseases and disorders to move well and the ability to progress strength and sport performance. At the dysfunctional level, striving for progression becomes a risk to pain and injury. This is the common mistake society makes jumping into training without looking at how they function to take the time to correct issues to prepare for strength. The NFL and NHL players, for example, do not just jump into training after taking 3 months off from playing. A habit changes quickly, as well as breathing and alignment instantly and requires training to reset them, much like the corporate officer worker sitting all day. Don't just move. Train your brain, your breathing and muscles to engage. Train slowly when trying to connect and integrate all the systems to perform together. When they are integrated you can then train speed, strength or power because you have the circuitry. Think, feel and blueprint through consistent repetition. Train your breath to stabilize and maintain alignment as well as using inhalation to produce power to be released through movement and to move. When movement is functional, you will intuitively breathe, stabilize and move well, without thinking. You will have created the functional system.

THE MOVEMENT ENCYCLOPEDIA

If you rather take a few movements at a time and perfect them first, it's ok. For example, take the lunge exercise and progress it through to the final advanced exercise over time. Instead of adding more exercises to your routine, add more range of motion and mobility to the exercise. The most important thing is to be aligned and functional. Don't compensate to move. It will steer you from the preventative and progressive path into compensation, dysfunction and pain. There is no rush to become advanced. Like I said before, anyone can move but how effective is your movement to produce strength, prevent pain and injury? Remember, you are not just moving, you are integrating the systems into one movement to get results: respiratory (breathing), musculoskeletal (muscles and joints) and nervous systems (the nerves). If it feels easy make sure you are applying all three.

Lunge Knee on Floor

- Get into a lunge position keeping the knee on the floor with the heel up and toes on the floor, not the ankle. Make sure the front foot is straight as well as the back heel keeping the stance close to the midline of the body.

- Maintain spinal alignment. Avoid leaning the spine forward. Focus on contracting the glute, stretching the hip flexor and bracing the abdominals as you lunge to the floor. This will provide the functional circuitry to maintain alignment and stability for the hip to stretch the hip flexor /quads into range of motion properly. If you stretch the hip flexor first without the glute contraction, you will be stretching misalignment and compensation and not producing balance, reciprocation and alignment. It will be harder to contract the glutes if the muscles are tight and inflexible. But you need the stability and balance of the hip through motion.

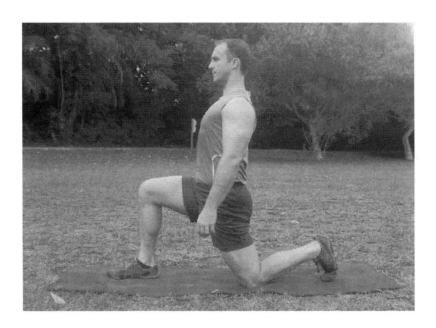

- First contract the glute and then breathe in through the nose bracing the abdominals moving the hip forward stretching the hip flexor.
- As you reach the tension barrier in the stretch, where motion stops, hold for 3 seconds the contraction of the glutes and brace the abdominals, then exhale hiss and lunge further. You will feel the range of motion increase.
- Breathe in again from the new position. Exhale hiss again for more motion. You will feel the inhalation load the stretch to power the exhalation. This is how the breathing cycle works.
- Perform for 3-5 breathing cycles and then switch sides.
- Keep your weight distributed to the front foot and leg, focusing on the big toe. This helps produce alignment for the knee. (If you push through the outside of the foot without using the big toe, your ankle will rotate out and imbalance the stability of the knee. Also, the big toe has a reflex to the glute medius muscle on the side of the hip to stabilize).
- Don't compensate to produce range of motion. You will produce more effective strength through the transference of the functional circuitry.

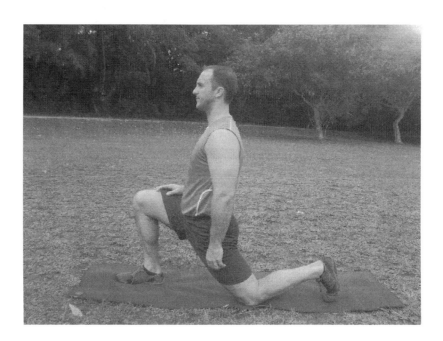

Lunge Knee on Floor Side Bend/Hyperextension

- With the knee on the floor, contract the glute, and stretch the hip flexor/quads.
- Breathe in lifting the arm opposite the leg forward straight into the air and bend the spine to the side contracting the obliques reaching the arm stretching the lats. With the leg forward knee, push the front foot into the floor as you side bend to activate the hip muscles.

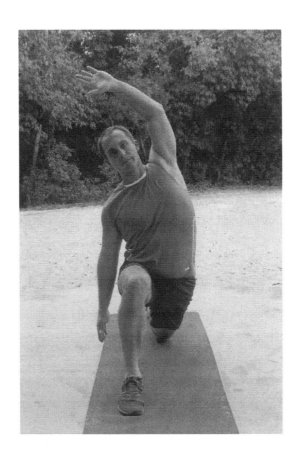

- Perform 3-5 breathing cycles in the side bend position and exhale hiss back to the center.
- Maintaining the glute contraction, breathe in, learn back and look up slowly hyperextending the spine contracting the spines muscles with the glutes. This will connect the hip with the spine.
- As you slowly lean back, focus on contracting the glute to maintain a foundation of support from the hips to transfer to the hyperextension of the spine. Keep the abdominals tight with the glutes and spine and don't let the stomach distend.
- Perform 3-5 breathing cycles in the hyperextension then exhale hiss back to center.
- Repeat the sequence from the start 3-5 times and then perform the other side.

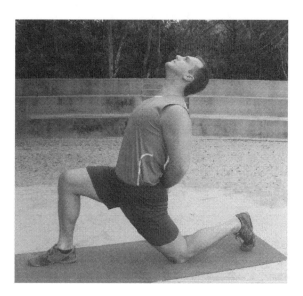

Remember, affecting the alignment and stability of a joint or muscle will improve ranges of motion. You will notice the side bend improving as well as the hyperextension that will transfer through other exercises.

Lunge Knee on Floor Flexion/ Rotation/ Hyperextension

- From the bottom lunge position with the knee on the floor, place the hands on the floor opposite side of the knee that is forward.
- Breathe in, contract the glute on the back leg stretching the hip flexor and perform 3-5 breathing cycles.

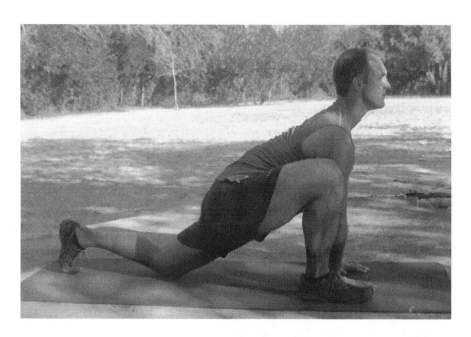

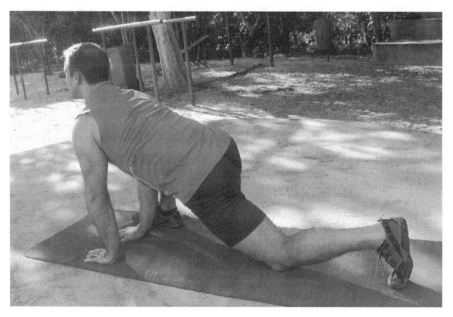

- Place the palm of your hand on your glute or the top of your wrist on your lower back. Breathe in stabilizing the abdominals and rotate the spine with the elbow in a chicken wing position. Rotating with the elbow helps the lat contract. As you contract the lat, focus on stabilizing the obliques on the opposite side focusing on the X movement pattern. The inhalation will help contract the lat and the oblique.

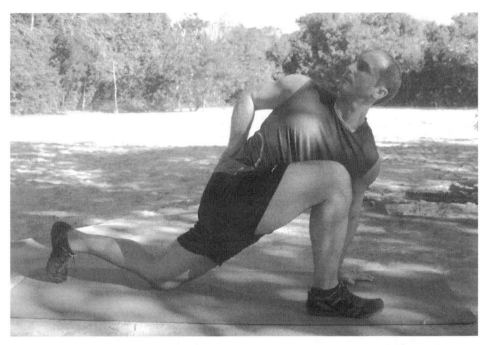

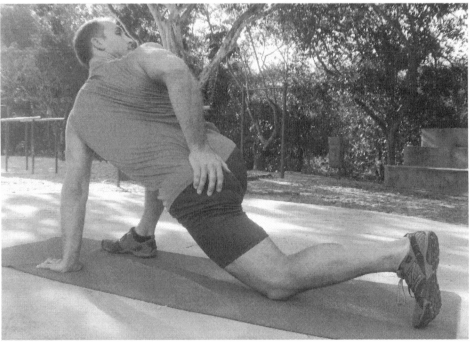

- Perform 3-5 breathing cycles at the same time rotating to improve more range of motion, linking the breath and motion together. Keep the abdominal brace active to avoid rounding the spine and glutes active to stabilize the hip and spine's position in the rotation. Think about breathing and alignment to create range of motion.
- You can also lift the arm up straight into the air from the bent arm position contracting the triceps, shoulders and lats.

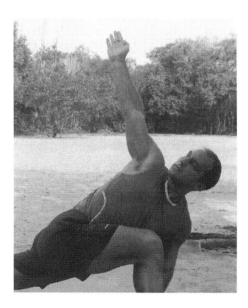

- After performing the breathing technique 3-5 times in the rotation, exhale hiss and move back to the neutral position from rotation.

- From the neutral position breathe in and hyperextend the spine. You can use the behind the arm technique or relax you hands in front of you.

- Perform for 3-5 breathing cycles in the hyperextension slowly contracting all the muscles to produce range of motion.

- Repeat the motions from the beginning 3-5 times and then switch sides.

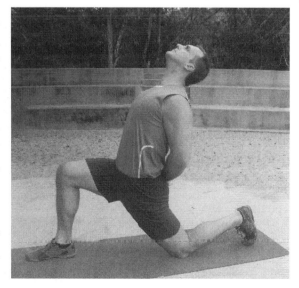

Lunge Knee off Floor Knee Bend Leg Extension

- Create a wide base lunge with the back leg knee bent off the floor contracting the glute.

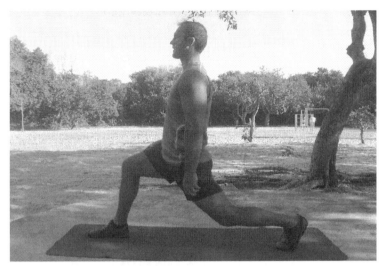

- Breathe in producing abdominal tension and at the same time contract the quads with the glute by straightening the leg, locking the knee. Don't lose the glute contraction when contracting the quads. The glute contracts first to maintain hip alignment and stability. Perform 3-5 breathing cycles lunging to the floor. On the exhale hiss, move back to the center position. Repeat and perform 3-5 times then switch sides.

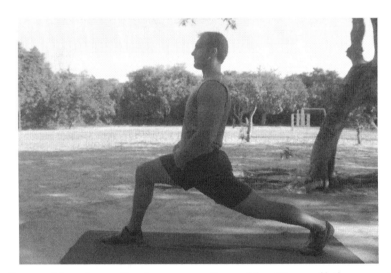

- On the forward leg, keep the knee over the ankle. Keep all the muscles contracted as you lunge and don't worry if the motion is big. You will need the strength of those muscles to contract in order to maintain hip alignment and produce range of motion. The more range the more stability you need.

Synergy Lunge- Hyperextension/ Neutral Rotation/ Flexion Rotation

- Perform in each position 3 -5 breathing cycles and the spine exercises with the leg straight in the knee lock position contracting the quads and glutes, like from the previous exercise. Repeat from the beginning 3-5 times then switch sides.

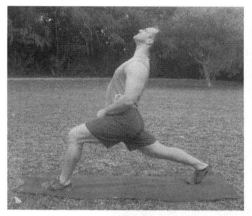 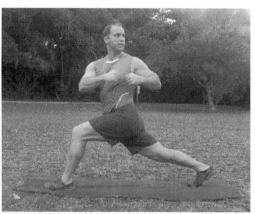

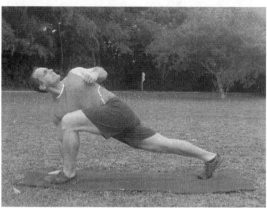

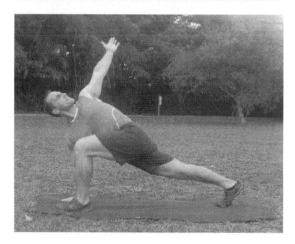

Top two photos from left to right -**Hyperextension and Neutral Rotation**
Bottom two photos from left to right- **Flexion Rotation with elbow and arm extension.**

Lying Down Knee Lift

- Contract the quads and the glutes on the straight leg and pull the toes toward the knee to stabilize the leg on the floor.
- Breathe in, brace the abdominals and lift one knee toward your chest (grab your knee with your hands on top and pull toward the chest if you need). Try not to let the lumbar round excessively and only lift as far as you functionally and comfortably can. Perform 3-5 breathing cycles pulling the knee up to the chest.
- Exhale hiss and lower the leg to the floor and perform the other side.
- Sometimes there is no mobility it is just an isometric static hold to develop stability first for mobility to happen, like developing the foundation first to build.

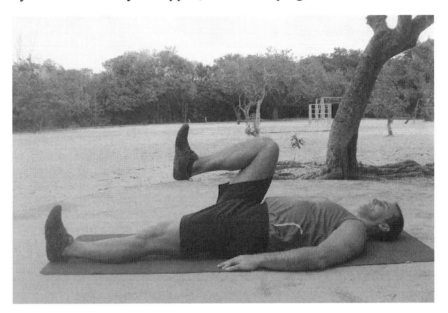

- Make sure when the knee is lifted that you track both feet and knees to the center.

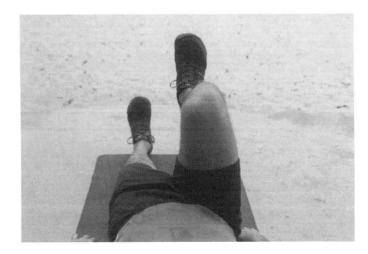

Side Leg Raise

- Lying on your side, breathe in and lift your leg up off the floor contracting the glute medius and TFL muscles on the side of the hip, the obliques by lifting the spine up slightly to bring power to the core as you left the leg, the ankle by pulling the toes toward the knee, and the quads by locking the knee. Perform 3-5 breathing cycles. On the exhale hiss lower the leg and lift and repeat 3-5 times and then switch sides.

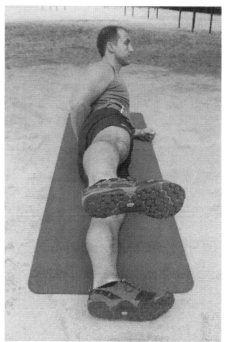

- Keep the foot straight, so you may have to fine-tune the rotators and glute medius muscles.

- If the muscles cramp or is difficult to maintain alignment, it is weak and can be the answer to issues with the ankle, knee and lower back as well as the spine.

- Bend your head to contract the muscles in the neck with the motion. You can place the arm behind the back or place the hand on top of the hip. I like the arm behind the back because it pulls the shoulder back and contracts the lat. Contracting the muscles helps create a blueprint for movement and the brain aligning the joints.

- You can move the leg front to back slightly contracting the muscles more thoroughly.

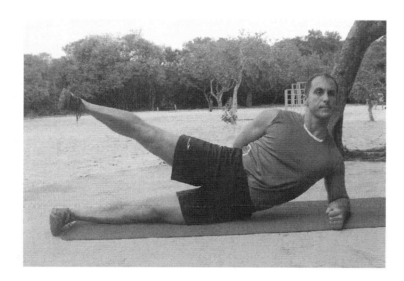

125

Side Leg Raise Knee Bend Leg Extension Kick

- From the side position place the top hand behind your back or put it on top of your hip. On the other arm, rest on your elbow engaging the oblique.
- Breathe in, lift the leg up and perform 3-5 breathing repetitions. On the inhalation, bend the knee toward the chest into a ninety-degree position and perform 3-5 breathing cycles pulling the knee to the chest. Keep the foot straight and toes slightly pulled toward the knee. Keeping the foot straight will fine-tune the rotators in the hip. So focus and be mindful.

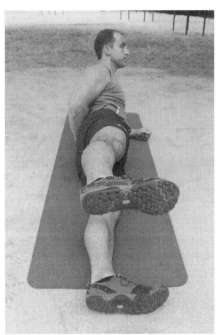 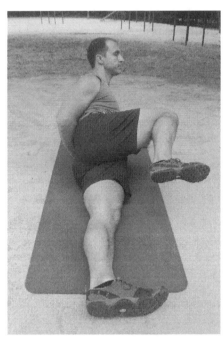

- On the exhale hiss, extend the leg, contracting the quads and the glutes while maintaining abdominal tension to the oblique. Perform 3-5 breathing cycles. Perform slowly contracting the muscles through movement. You will feel the inhalation load the stretch and range of motion. Repeat from the start for 3-5 times.

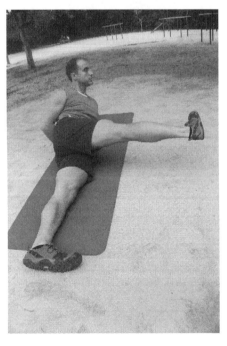

Side Leg Raise Knee Bend Leg Extension Kick Leg Curl

- From the side position, breathe in lift the leg up to the center contracting the glute medius, Perform 3-5 breathing cycles from this position.
- Breathe in and bend the knee up. Perform 3-5 breathing cycles pulling the knee to the chest.
- Exhale hiss and extend the leg. Perform 3-5 breathing cycles pulling the toes toward the knee and contracting the quads.

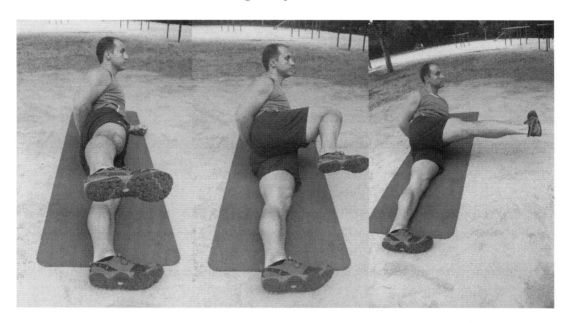

- Breathe in and curl the leg back contracting the hamstrings and glutes. Perform 3-5 breathing cycles curling the leg. Exhale hiss and move the leg back to the center and repeat from the beginning 3-5 times and then switch sides.

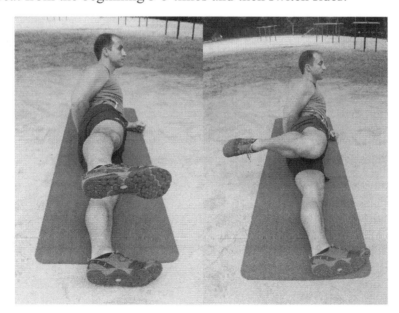

- You should notice that there is more range from the joint or the movement is easier in the second or third breathing cycle. Maintain alignment from the shoulder to the hip to the ankle. Maintain the abdominal brace to maintain lumbar stability and overall stability to transfer through the motion. Breathing in braces and prevents hyperextension especially when curling the leg. If you arch or round the spine, you will lose alignment and decrease muscle stability. Keep the toes slightly pulled toward the knee.

Lying Down Side Bend Leg Scissor Hip Rotation

- Lying on your back move your legs into an open scissors position. You should feel the muscles on the side of the hips contract. If they cramp move the legs slightly closer, you went to far.
- Breathe in and bend your spine to the left to contract the oblique and lat, the quads and glutes on **both legs** and slightly pull the toes toward the knees.
- Perform 3-5 breathing cycles along with contracting the muscles.
- Exhale hiss, relax and move the spine back to the center.
- Breathe in and bend your spine to the right side contracting the oblique, lat, the quads and glutes on **both legs** and slightly pull the toes toward the knees. Perform for 3-5 breathing cycles. Repeat alternating side to side 3-5 times. See if more range of motion appears or if the position becomes easier to maintain.

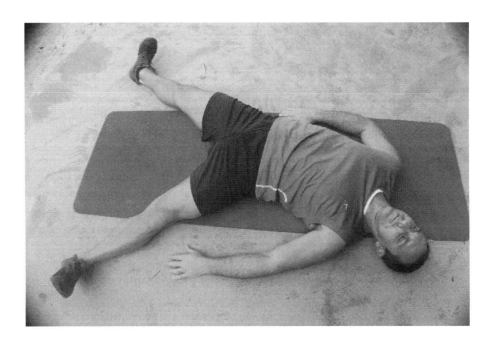

Leg Scissors Off Floor

- Breathe in and lift your legs off the floor. Perform 3-5 breathing cycles stabilizing the legs off the floor.

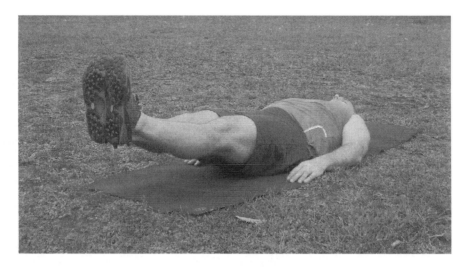

- Exhale hiss and open the legs into a scissor position.
- When you open the legs rotate the hips and feet. Perform 3-5 breathing cycles holding the position and move the legs back together.
- Repeat 3-5 times.

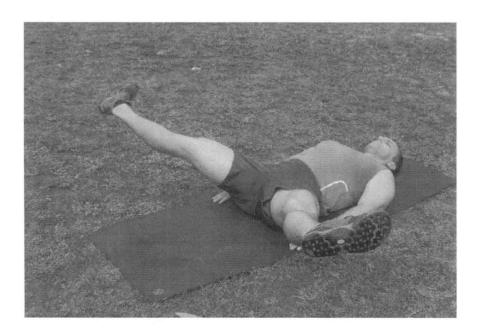

Single Leg Hip Hinge

- Place one-foot forward and one back. Keep the back leg straight and the front leg knee slightly bent. The front leg will do the work.

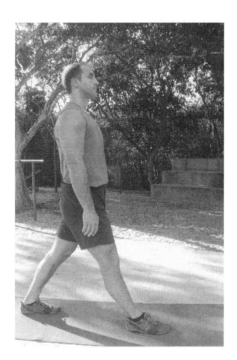 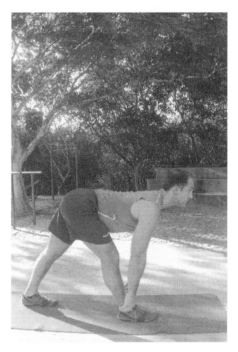

- Hinge over as far as you can possible without losing spinal alignment.

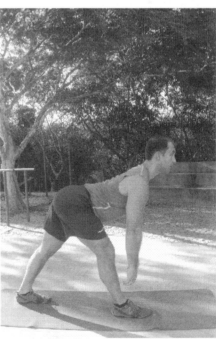

- From the hip hinge position, note that your spine may not be as low as the photo above, it is ok. Find a comfortable position that maintains alignment.

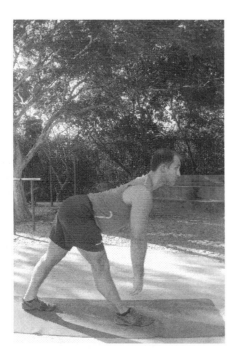 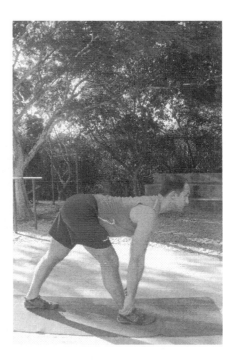

- From the hip hinge position, straighten the leg by contracting the quads to stretch the hamstrings. Perform 3-5 breathing cycles stretching the hamstring. Focus on lifting the hips up. You will feel the inhalation load the stretch to power the exhalation.
- Keep the weight distributed through the whole foot. Make sure you place the weight onto the big toe. It will make a big difference in what you feel in the movement. You will feel the glute medius activate in the hip and the knee will track properly.
- Perform the other side.

Hip Hinge Close Stance Squat Leg Extension

- Stand with your feet close together and knees slightly bent.
- Breathe in and slowly squat keeping the knees center and the heels on the ground placing weight through the whole foot using the big toe. This will help the knees track in the center and activate glute medius on the side of the hip as you squat.
- Hold the squat position for 3-5 breathing cycles and see if more mobility happens or feels easier to maintain the position.

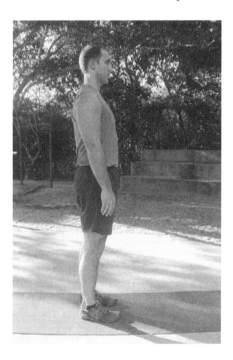 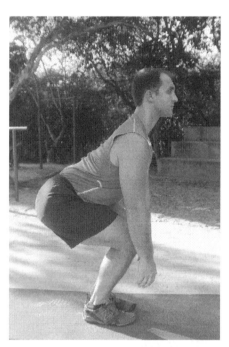

- Exhale hiss and straighten the legs by contracting the quads. Focus on lifting the hips up and straightening the spine. Hold the position for 3-5 breathing cycles. Repeat each motion 3-5 times.
- Don't force. Move into the best position you can. Keep your legs straight and focus on the big toe back to the heel and inside of the foot.
- You can shift your weight back and forth from the toes to the heels to stabilize and stretch different muscles.

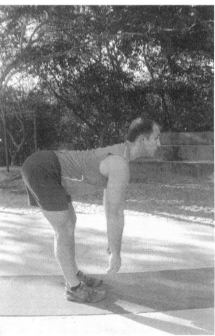

Lying Down Knee Bend Leg Extension

- Lying on your back breathe in bracing your abdominals and lift your knee to your stomach. (On the straight leg keep the toes straight and slightly pulled toward the knee contracting the quads and the glute. What you do on the straight leg affects the knee lift). Perform for 3-5 breathing cycles pulling the knee up.

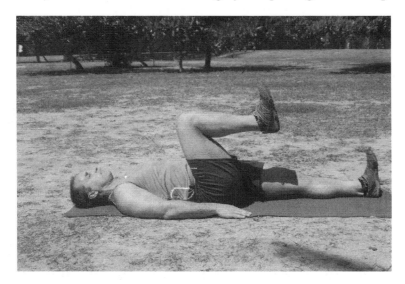

- Exhale hiss and straighten the leg contracting the quads pulling the toes down toward the knee to stretch the hamstrings. Remember, the hiss activates and stabilizes the abdominals. When you straighten the leg up, maintain the glute and quad contraction to the leg on the floor and keep the foot straight preventing the foot and hip from rotating. It makes a difference in the movement.
- Perform for 3-5 breathing cycles in the straight leg position, bracing, contracting and stretching. Repeat each motion 3-5 times and then switch sides.

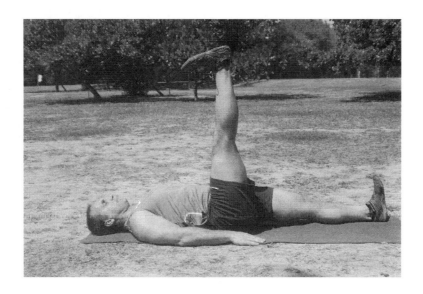

133

Hip Hinge Reach Back Y

- Breathe in create abdominal stability and move the hips into the hinge position. Stretch the hamstrings and contract the quads. You can keep the knees slightly bent as well. Perform 3-5 breathing cycles in this position.

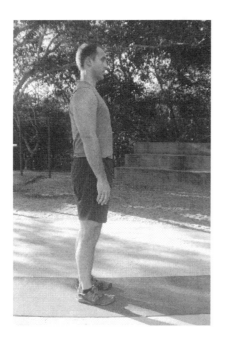 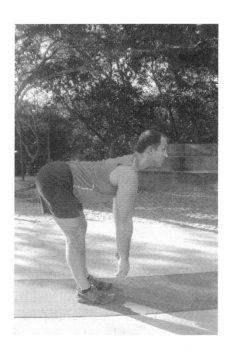

- On the inhalation, reach your arms back. You can slightly hyperextending your spine (photo to the right) or keep the spine straight (photo **top** right). When reaching back lift the arms up to contract the triceps, lats and shoulders. When you have position, push the hands toward each other. Perform 3-5 breathing cycles reaching the arms back.

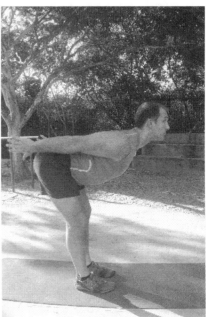

- On the exhale hiss reach your arms into a Y position. Maintaining abdominal tension when reaching your arms forward into a Y contracting the lats, shoulders and triceps (bottom photo) straightening the spine.
- When you move the arms forward keep the spine flat not arched or rounded. Use the pressure in the abdominals and hamstrings tension to reach through the arms. Keep the big toe active and not just lean back into the heels of the feet.
- Perform 3-5 breathing cycles in the Y position. Repeat the sequence 3-5 times.

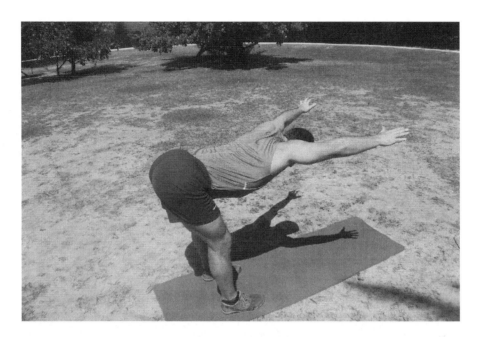

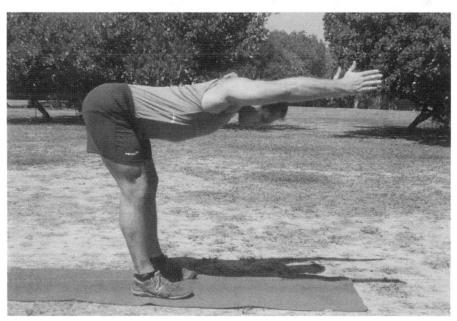

Hip Hinge Lat Rotation Windmill

- From the hip hinge position, breathe in and rotate the spine reaching the elbow back contracting the lat and the other arm reaching across the body activating the obliques. One leg will be straight contracting the quads and on the other leg the knee will be slightly bent pushing the foot into the ground.
- Contract the obliques, shoulders, back, quads and biceps for 3-5 breathing cycles rotating the spine and see if more range opens. Repeat alternating side to side 3-5 times on each side. It is important that you maintain the abdominal/spine stability keeping the spine straight.

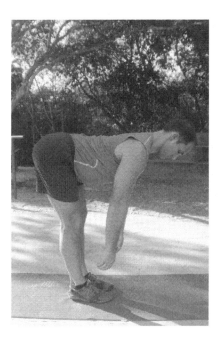 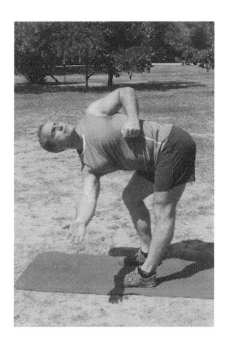

- Once you have good rotation you can extend the arm contracting the triceps, the lats and back of the shoulders.

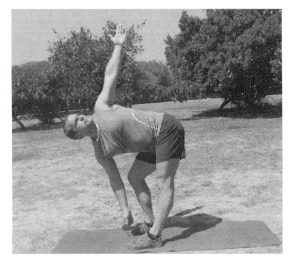

Single Leg Frog

- Face down on your forearms, bring one knee up into a 90 degree position.
- On the straight leg, contract the quads and the glutes. This will bring the knee slightly off the floor. Contracting and stabilizing the muscles on the straight leg makes the bent leg up, move properly from alignment and stability.
- With the leg that has the knee up, breathe in bracing the abdominals and isometrically push the knee into the floor. Try to flatten the inner thigh on the floor. Perform for 3-5 breathing cycles.
  .

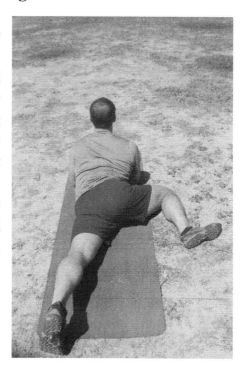

- Keep the shoulders square and the spine aligned. Don't compensate the spine to lift the knee up. Start with it lower if needed. Feel for differences on the left and right sides.
- Exhale hiss and perform the other side.

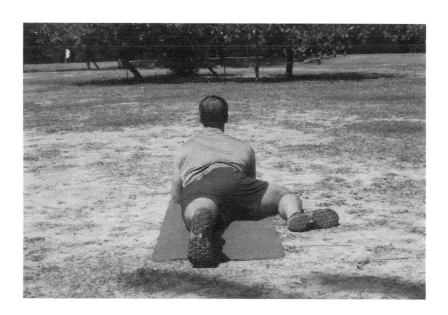

Single Leg Frog Leg Extension

- Face down on your forearms, bring one knee up into a 90 degree position.
- On the straight leg, contract the quads and the glutes. This will bring the knee slightly off the floor. Contracting and stabilizing the muscles on the straight leg makes the bent leg up move properly from alignment and stability.

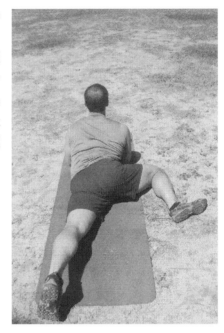

- Extend the bent knee leg straight. Once the leg is extended contract the quads to feel the muscles of the hip react and contract and slightly pull the toes toward the knee.
- Perform 3-5 breathing cycles and perform the other side.

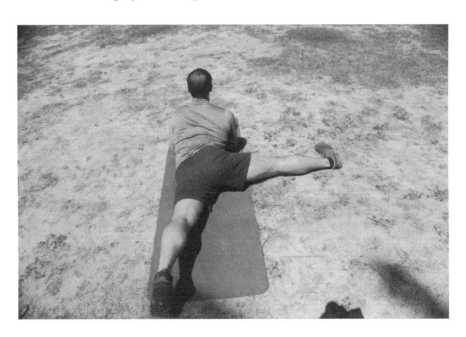

Frog

- Spread your knees open stretching the inner thighs, keeping the ankles open to the floor (Photo 1) or turning your feet out (Photo 2).

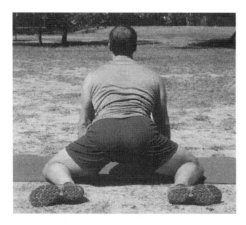 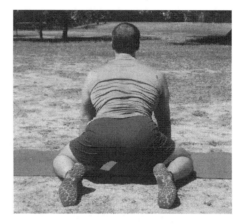

- Breathe in pushing your hands into the floor and push your hips back contracting the abs, shoulders, lats, triceps and the hip muscles. Perform 3-5 breathing cycles pushing the hips into the sit back position. (Photo 1- Left)

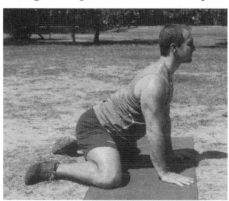 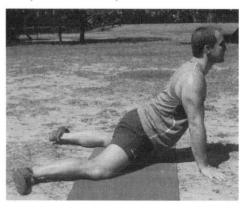

- On the exhalation hiss and walk you hands out in front of you extending your legs. Maintain the brace and a straight spine without hyperextending your lower back. You will feel the stretch of the inner thigh and glute medius contraction. Perform 3- 5 breathing cycles in the extended position. (Photo 2-Right)

- On the inhalation, walk the hands back slowly to sit toward your heels again. (Photo 1- above) Keep moving back to where you feel the hands pushing into the floor, pushing the hips toward the heels like the starting position. Maintain the core and spinal alignment for optimal flexibility to develop and occur.

- **OPTIONAL: If you choose exhale hiss slowly and rotate one hip up by bringing one foot off the floor. Breathe in and lower it.**

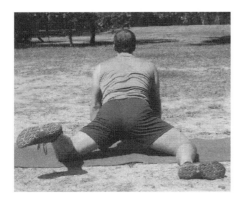 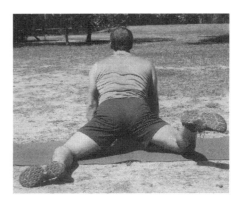

Lying Down Knee Bend/ Leg Extension/ Hip Rotation/ Lateral Drop

- Keep the leg and foot on the floor straight, contracting the glute and quads to create the foundation of alignment and stability in the movement.

- Breathe in tightening the abdominals and lift the knee up toward the chest for 3-5 breathing cycles.

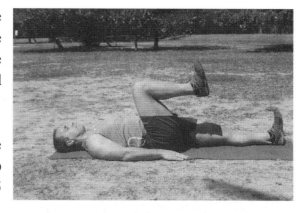

- Exhale hiss and extend the leg up contracting the quads, slightly pulling the toes down toward the knee to stretch the hamstrings for 3-5 breathing cycles.

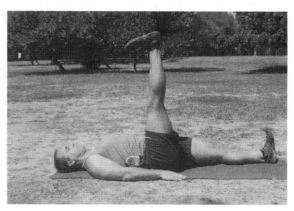

- Then, breathe in, rotate the foot and hip and move the leg laterally contracting the glute medius stretching the adductor. Keep the toes pulled slightly toward the knee to stretch the hamstring and contract the quads. Perform for 3-5 breathing cycles.

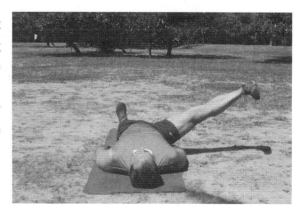

- Make sure you contract the glutes and quads on the straight leg on the floor for stability to move the other leg.

Alternate Lateral Squat

- Assume a mid squat position with the feet straight or slightly turned out. Breathe in and squat to one side keeping the foot flat on the floor and the knee over the big toe.
- Feel the shin muscles contract and the calf muscles stretch. You will feel the glute medius on the side of the hip contract as well.
- On the stretched leg, try to contract the quads and slightly pull the toes toward the knee. Also try to slightly rotate the foot back to activate the hip stabilizers.
- Hold the bottom position and perform 3 to 5 breathing cycles and return to the start position and perform the other side, alternating side-to-side.
- Use your hands for balance on the ground. Only go as far as you are comfortable. You don't have to go all the way to the floor.

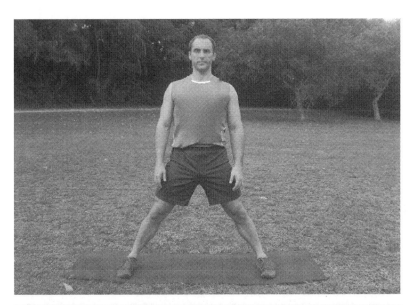

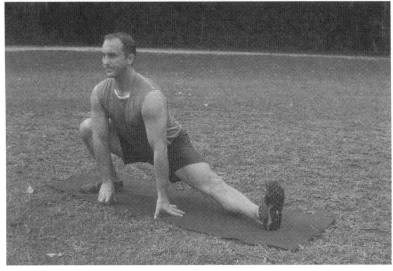

Hip Bridge

- Lying on the floor with the knees up and feet flat, keep the knees less than shoulder width apart. You should have enough space for a fist or less, between the knees. I like to push the knees together to contract the adductors with the glutes.

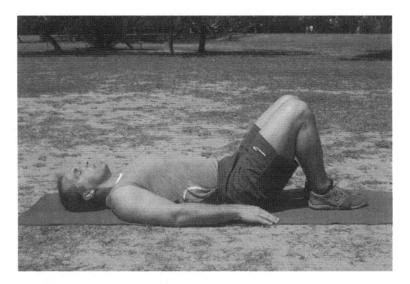

- Breathe in and lift the hips up into the air. Push your feet into the floor to lift the hips high contracting the glutes, hamstrings and abdominals. Perform 3-5 breathing cycles along with pushing the feet into the floor and hips up. Keep the hips active by pushing through the feet. Keep the knees tracked in the center.

- The bracing breath is important in the hip bridge because it will prevent excessive lumbar extension and provide more stability to the lumbar. You can add more tension by pushing your hands into the floor to contract the lats, shoulders and triceps. Exhale hiss and lower the hips down.

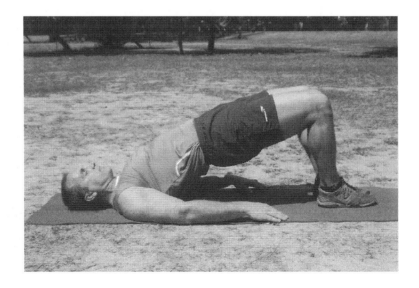

Single Leg Hip Bridge Knee Bend

- Laying on your back with your knees bent and feet flat on the floor. Breathe in and lift your hips up into the air contracting the glutes. This will be the start position.

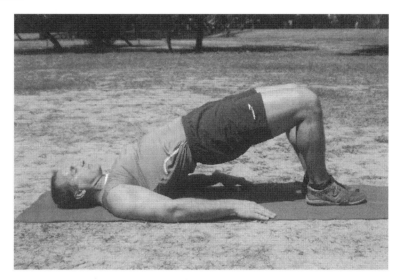

- On the same inhalation, lifting one knee toward the chest, perform 3 -5 breathing cycles and then perform the other side.
- The leg and foot you are hip bridging with is active pushing the hips up, contracting the glutes, stabilizing the hips off the floor. Don't let the hips sag.
- Push the whole foot into the floor at the same time you pull the knee actively toward the chest. The leg-bridging knee should be tracking in the center, not tracking away or inward of the body. Stabilize the position.

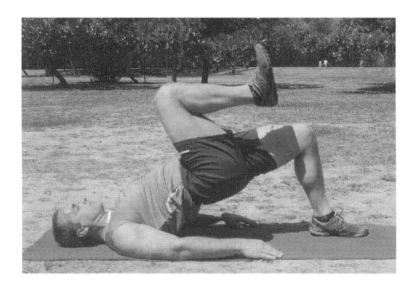

Single Leg Hip Bridge Knee Bend Lever

- Lay on your back with your knees bent and feet flat on the floor and lift the hips up into the air. This it the start position.

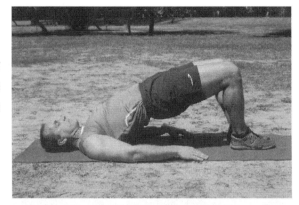

- Breathe in and lift the knee up toward the chest for 3-5 breathing cycles at the same time pulling the knee toward the chest.

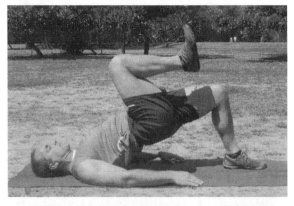

- Exhale hiss and extend the leg into a lever contracting the quads and pulling the toes toward the knee to stretch the hamstrings. Perform for 3-5 breathing cycles.

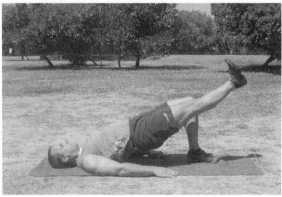

- Breathe in and bend the knee again back toward the chest (photo 2) and switch sides. Perform 3-5 times in each position.

Single Leg Hip Bridge Knee Bend Lever Leg Extension

- Breathe in and lift the hips up, bringing the knee toward the chest. Perform 3-5 breathing cycles.

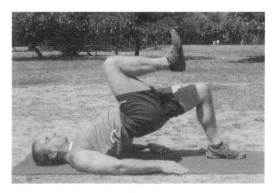

- Exhale hiss and lever the leg contracting the quads slightly pulling the toes toward knee for 3-5 breathing cycles.

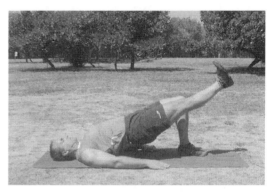

- Exhale hiss and lift the leg up, maintaining the contraction of the quads, pulling the toes toward the knee when you extend the leg straight up.

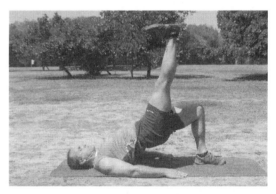

- Once the leg is in position, perform 3-5 breathing cycles.

- Repeat for all the movements and breathing cycles 3 to 5 times then switch legs.

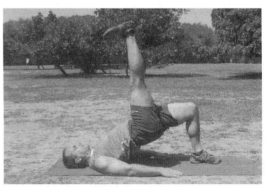

Single Leg Hip Bridge Lever Leg Extension Lateral Drop

- Breathe in and bend the knee up toward the chest. Perform 3-5 breathing cycles. In each position, focus on the inhalation for contraction and exhalation for stretch and range of motion.

- Exhale hiss and lever the leg contracting the quads and slightly pulling the toes toward the knee for 3-5 breathing cycles.

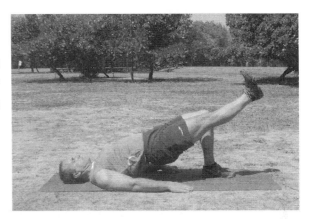

- Breathe in and extend the leg up contracting the quads slightly pulling the toes toward the knee stretching the hamstrings for 3-5 breathing cycles.

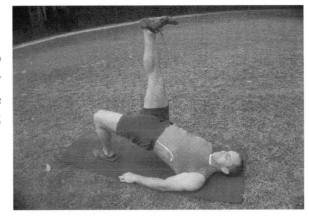

- Exhale hiss and lower the leg to the side contracting the quads and glute medius, slightly pulling the toes toward the knee to stretch the hamstrings and inner thigh. Perform for 3-5 breathing cycles. Repeat the sequence from the beginning 3-5 times.

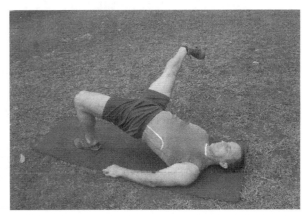

Face Down Knee Lock Leg Scissors

- Lying on your stomach resting on your elbows, move your legs into a scissor position. Keep the knees relaxed touching the floor and the feet straight.

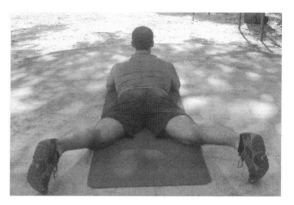

- Breathe in contracting the quads and the glutes.

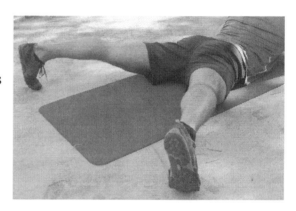

- Exhale hiss and see if the position is more comfortable or if you can scissor a little further. If the muscles cramp they are weak. Continue the movement over time until the cramping stops and the muscle becomes stronger.

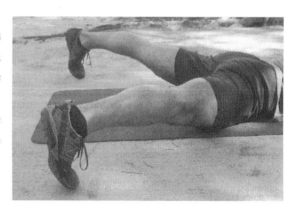

- When contracting the glutes and quads, you will feel the lower back muscles contract.
- Perform for 3-5 breathing cycles.

Face Down Knee Touch Leg Curl Lift Leg Extension

- Lying face down resting on your elbows, breathe in and lift the knees and the lower part of the legs and feet off the floor. Hold for 3-5 breathing cycles.

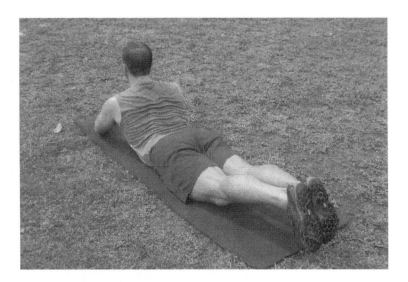

- On the exhale hiss curl your legs, keeping the feet straight. Touch your knees together or keep them about a fist width apart. Hold the position and perform 3-5 breathing cycles. Repeat 3-5 times, extending and curling the legs with the breathing cycles 3-5 times in each motion.
- When you breathe in focus on pushing through your abdominals to lift. As you lift, push the knees together or keep them slightly apart, this will activate the inner thigh muscles, hip muscles, abdominals and lower back muscles all together.

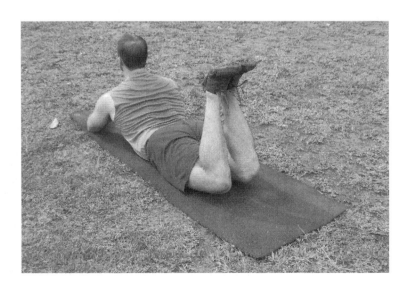

Face Down Knee Touch Leg Curl Lift Leg Extension Scissor

- Lying face down resting on your elbows, curl your legs keeping the feet straight. Touch your knees together or keep them a fist width apart. Perform 3-5 breathing cycles in this position.

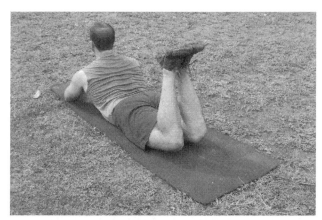

- Breathe in and lift the knees, lower part of the legs and feet off the floor. Focus on pushing through your abdominal pressure to lift. Perform for 3-5 breathing cycles.

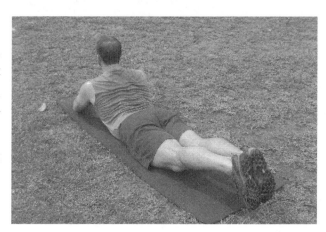

- Exhale hiss and extend your legs into a scissor position contracting the quads and glutes. Perform for 3-5 breathing cycles holding the position. Breathe in and straighten the legs.

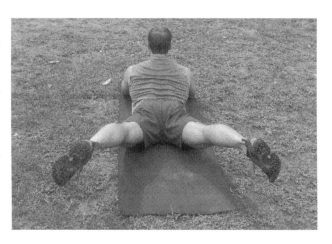

- Repeat 3-5 times the sequence of motions.

Face Down Leg Scissors Off Floor

- Breathe in and lift your legs off the floor with the knees touching for 3-5 breathing cycles.

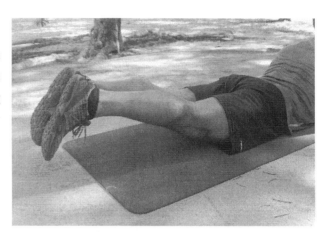

- Exhale his separating the legs rotating the feet and the hips. As you rotate the feet and the hips you will feel the glute medius contract.

- Maintain the buttock contraction as you scissor the legs open.

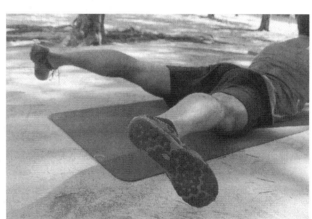

- Perform 3-5 breathing cycles in the extended position contracting the muscles.

- Breathe in and bring the legs back together touching the knees.

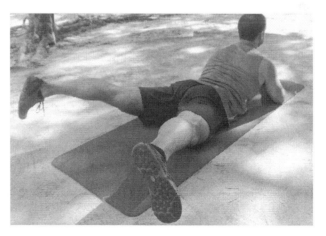

- Repeat 3-5 times in each position

Face Down Scorpion Leg Scissor

- Laying face down on your elbows, breathe in, curl your leg and lift your knee and foot up and across the body. You will lift your hip up off the floor as well. Lifting the hip causes other muscles to contract. When you lift the leg and hip, keep the spine aligned. As you lift the leg keep the abdominals tight from the inhalation. Perform 3-5 breathing cycles.

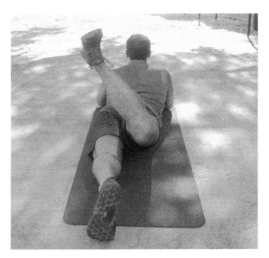

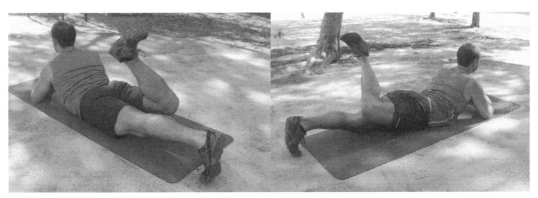

- Don't compensate the spines alignment to create range of motion. With the straight leg on the floor, contract the quads and glutes to maintain stability in the movement. It is important to create the stability for range of motion to move.

- Exhale hiss, straighten the leg contracting the quads, glutes and slightly pointing the toes toward the knee and scissor the leg away from the body contracting the glute medius. Perform for 3-5 breathing cycles in that position.

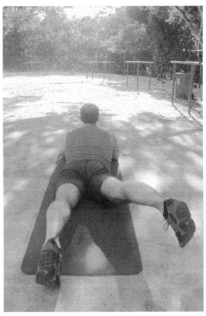

- You will feel the lower back muscles and obliques when scissoring the leg. By contracting the quads you will transfer tension to the lumbar and gluteal muscles. Breathe in bring the leg back into the scorpion. Repeat the motions 3-5 times.

Face Down Scorpion Leg Scissor Side Bend

- From the face down position breathe in and lift the leg up into scorpion position. Perform 3-5 breathing cycles holding, contracting and stabilizing the position.

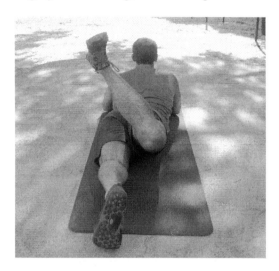

- Exhale hiss, straighten the leg contracting the quads and glutes and move the leg away from the body into a scissor position off the floor. With the upper body, push your hand into the floor and bend to the side contracting the lats and the obliques on the same side of the leg scissor. Perform 3-5 breathing cycles contracting all the muscles in this position. Keep the quads and glutes contracted in the scissor to feel the lower back stabilize. With the straight leg on the floor, contract the quads and glutes to transfer stability through the movement. Breathe in and bring the leg back to the center. Repeat 3-5 times.

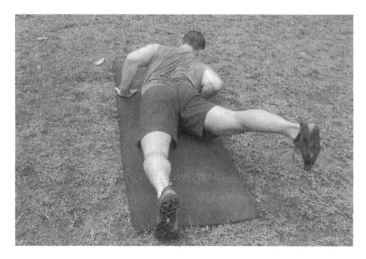

Face Down Windmill

- From face down position move your legs into a scissor position contracting the glutes and quads.

- Breathe in and lift yourself up reaching your arms back. You don't need to lift so high. Just lift to a point where the bottom of the rib cage and top of the abdominals are still on the floor. Hold and perform 3-5 breathing cycles.

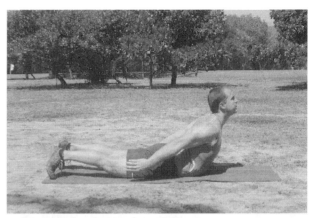

- Exhale hiss reaching one arm forward and the other back. When you reach back, contract the lats, shoulders and triceps. Keep the glutes and quads contracted. Don't force the rotation. Hold and perform 3-5 breathing cycles.

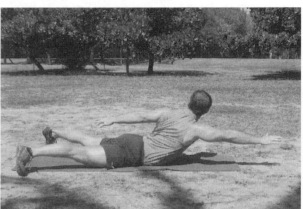

- Exhale hiss, switching sides reaching the other arm forward for 3-5 breathing cycles. Breathe in back to center. Repeat 3-5 times alternating side to side.

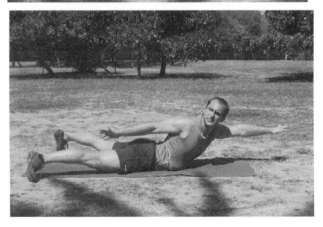

Face Down Leg Lifts

- Laying face down, breathe in and push your hands into the floor to contract your triceps and lat's.

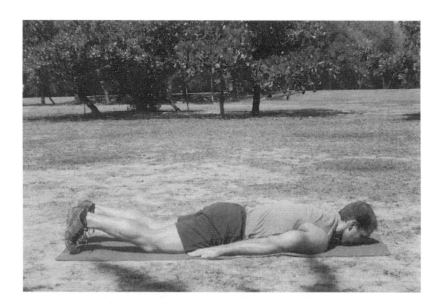

- Exhale hiss and lift your legs up into the air pushing through your hands. Use the pressure from the breath to produce a fulcrum for the abdominals. Hold for 3-5 breathing cycles.

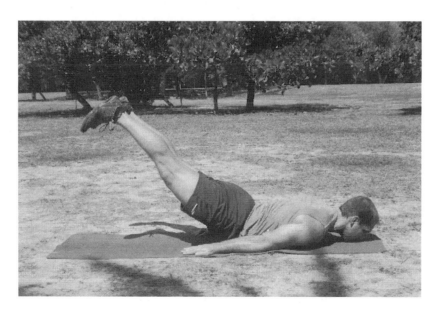

- As you lift your legs, contract your glues, quads and lats. Use your breath and abdominal tension as a fulcrum. On the exhale hiss, lower down. Repeat 3- 5 times.

Standing Knee Raise

- The standing knee raise is the same as the Lying Down Isometric Knee Lift except for standing, using your alignment and stability.

- Breathe in brace the abdominals, (the breathing can either way breathe in exhale and then lift the knee) contract the glutes and quads on the standing leg to preserve alignment and stability for the hip lifting the knee. Lift the knee only as high as you can without compensation. Keep the spine straight not rounded. Perform 3-5 breathing cycles at the same time lifting the knee, stabilizing and contracting the glutes on the straight leg.

- Perform 3-5 repetitions and then the other side.

- You can use added resistance by pressing your hand on your knee when lifting it up.This exercise is great for developing balance, coordination and synchronization for stability and mobility through movement.

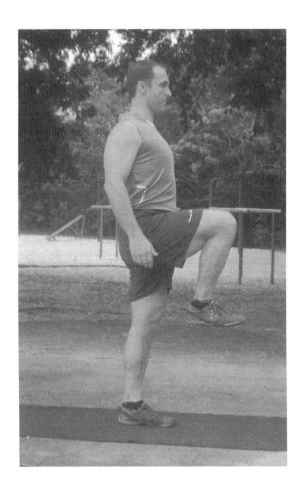

Seated Leg Extension (Sitters Routine)

- From a sitting position roll the pelvis forward and keep the spine tall maintaining the ear, shoulder and hip alignment.
- Breathe in and extend the leg straight out in front contracting the quads. Once the leg is in the extended position, slowly and slightly pull the toes back toward the knee. Keep the foot at a 90-degree angle position. When lifting the leg, don't let the spine lean back or round forward. Stabilize the abdominals and lift the leg. Hold and perform for 3-5 breathing cycles with the leg in the extended position. You will feel the quads contract, hamstrings stretch and abdominals, obliques and lumbar stabilize.
- Perform the other side alternating back and forth for 3-5 times.

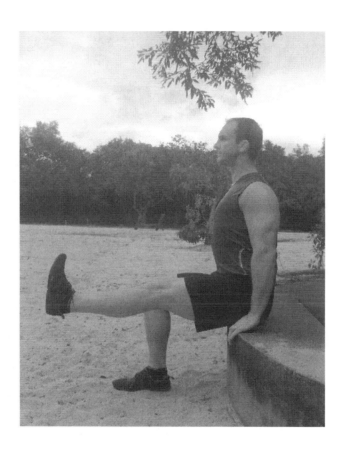

Seated Leg Extension Hip Rotation

- From the seated position, sit up straight. Breathe in and with one leg extend the leg contracting the quads. Once the leg is extended, slightly pull the toes toward the knee. When you extend the leg, don't round the spine keep the spine straight stabilizing the abdominals to stabilize the force generated from the leg. Perform 3-5 breathing cycles.
- Rotate the foot inward and perform 3-5 breathing cycles and then exhale hiss back to center.
- Breathe in and rotate the foot away from the body. Perform 3-5 breathing cycles, exhale hiss and rotate back to center. Keep the quads contracted as you rotate the hip.

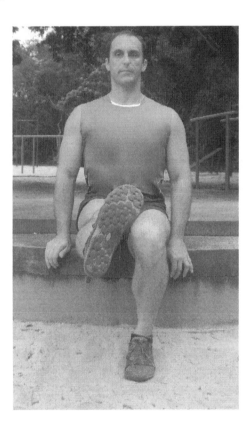 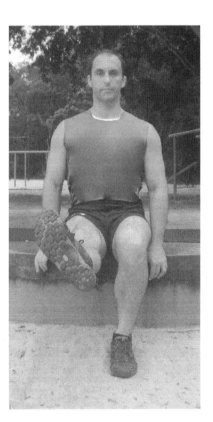

Seated Flexion Hyperextension

- Sitting in a chair keep the hips rolled forward.
- Breathe in bracing the abdominals as you round the spine forward. Don't force a stretch. If you do it correct you wont feel a stretch, just stabilization Perform 3-5 breathing. Exhale hiss back to the center.
- Breathe in keeping the hips rolled forward and hyperextend the spine and neck looking up contracting the back muscles. Focus on the inhalation and the contraction of muscles. Keep the abdominals tight and braced not distended. Perform 3-5 breathing cycles. Exhale hiss back to the center. Perform slowly, focusing on breathing, the abdominals and spine for stability.
- Repeat 3-5 times.

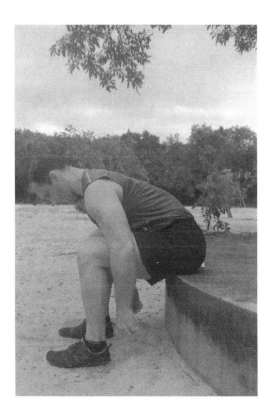 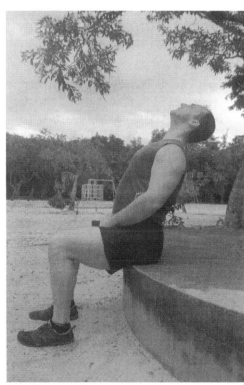

Seated Side Bend One Arm Reach

- From the seated position, reach one arm up above your head. Breathe in and bend to the side. Contract the lat and oblique on the side that the arm is down and stretch the lat on the reaching arm. Perform 3-5 breathing cycles.
- Exhale hiss back to center and perform the other side. Lift the other arm up breathe in and bend. Perform 3-5 breathing cycles. Exhale hiss back to center.
- Perform 3-5 times alternating side to side for each rep.
- You can use a straight or bent arm in the reach.

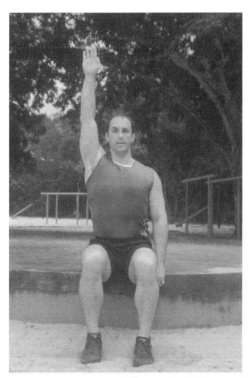 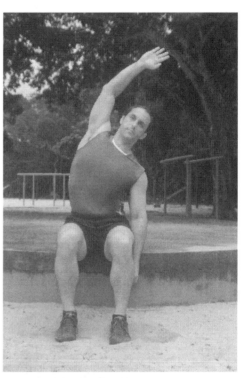

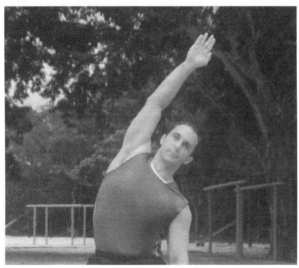

Seated Lat Rotation

- Sitting in a chair bring your arms into a 90-degree position.
- Breathe in and rotate the head and spine to one side contracting the neck, shoulder, lat and the oblique. As you rotate, move the elbow in the rotation toward the spine. Focus on contracting the lats to rotate the spine. Perform 3-5 breathing in the rotation. Exhale hiss back to center. Focus on the X Movement Pattern (right oblique, left lat and shoulder and vise versa). Perform the other side.
- Repeat 3-5 times alternating back and forth to each side for balance.

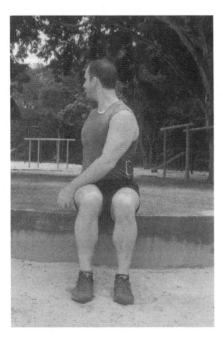 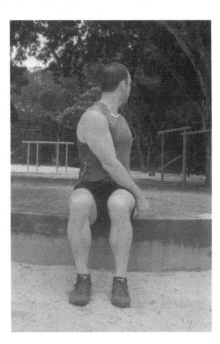

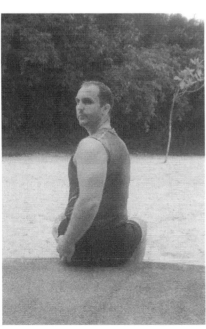 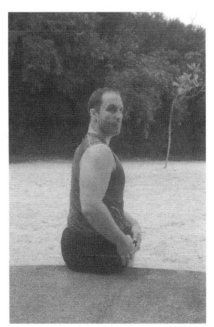

Seated Side Bend Lat Rotation

- Sitting in a chair reach your arm straight up in the air. Perform 3-5 breathing cycles as you reach the arm up.
- Breathe in and bend to the side. Perform 3-5 breathing cycles bending to the side.
- Exhale hiss back to center. Bring the arm down, breathe in and rotate. Perform 3-5 breathing cycles as you rotate.
- Exhale hiss back to center and perform the other side. Repeat 3-5 times.

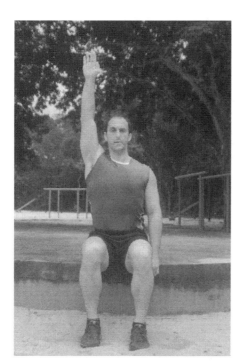 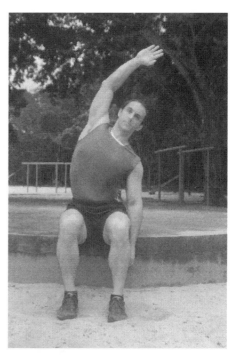

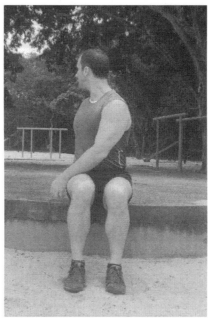

Standing Flexion Hyperextension

- From a standing position with feet shoulder width apart and feet straight, breathe in and slowly roll down to the ground. Keep the abdominals tight to transfer it to the spine. Contract the quads. Don't try to stretch the spine. Let it naturally round into flexion around the abdominal tension and pressure without bending it excessively. Perform 3-5 breathing cycles and exhale hiss back to the center.

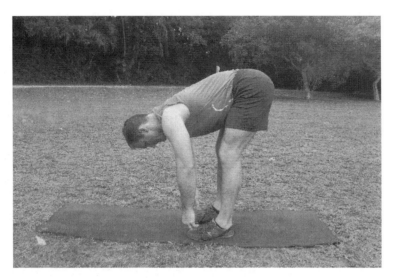

- From the center breathe in again keeping the abdominals tight and hyperextend the spine contracting the quads, glutes and spine muscles looking up and back. Lift the chest and pull the shoulders back. Rolling the shoulders back activates more abdominal stability than if the shoulders are forward. Focus on the inhalation and the contraction of muscles. Keep the abdominals tight and braced not distended. Perform 3-5 breathing cycles then exhale hiss back to the center. Perform slowly, focusing on breathing, the abdominals and spine for stability. Repeat 3- 5 times.

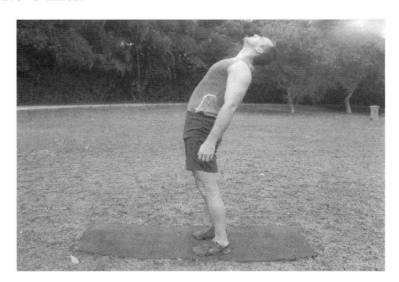

Standing Side Bend One Arm Reach

- From the standing position spread the feet shoulder width apart, contract the glutes and quads and breathe in reaching one arm up above your head bending to the side.

- Contract the lat and oblique on the side the arm is down and stretch on the arm that is up. Keep the abdominals, obliques, lats and glutes tight bending from this platform. Continue for 3-5 breathing cycles in the side bend. On the last exhale move back to the center. Perform the other side. Alternate side to side 3-5 times on each side.

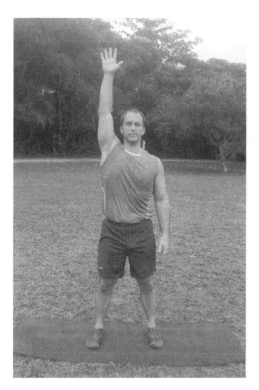 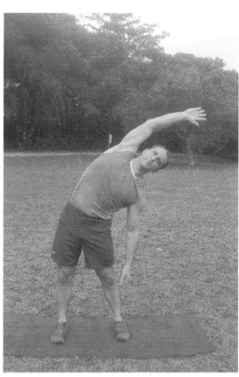

Standing Lat Rotation

- From the standing position with feet shoulder width apart contract the quads and glutes. This will help stabilize the hips in the rotation.
- Bring your arms up into a 90-degree position or keep by your side.
- Breathe in and rotate the head and spine to one side contracting the neck, shoulder, lat and the oblique. As you rotate move the elbow in the rotation toward the spine. Focus on contracting the lats to rotate the spine. Perform 3-5 breathing cycles in the rotation. Focus on the X Movement Pattern (right oblique, left lat and shoulder and vise versa). Perform the other side. Repeat 3-5 times alternating side to side.

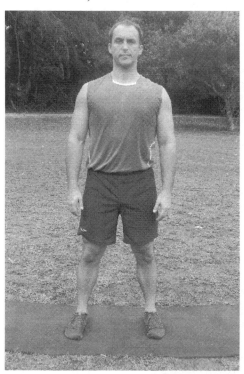 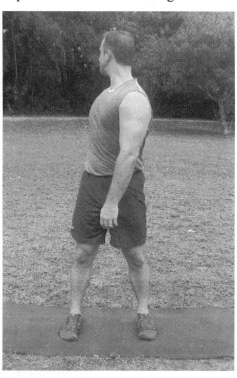

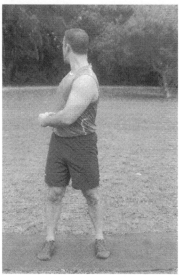

Low Kneeing Flexion Extension

- On your knees sitting back on your heels, breathe in and extend the spine from the flexion position. Perform 3-5 breathing cycles in the flexion position.
- Exhale hiss and extend your spine. Hold the extension and perform 3- 5 breathing cycles. Repeat 3-5 times.

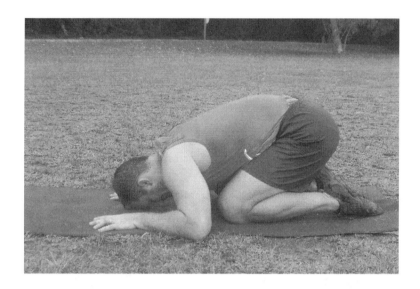

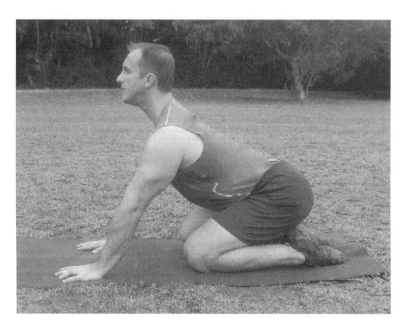

Low Kneeling Flexion High Kneeling Hyperextension

- Kneeling on the floor, sit back on your heels. Breathe in stabilizing and bracing the abdominals and push your hands into the floor to activate the back muscles, also push your hips back into your heels. Perform for 3-5 breathing cycles. On the last exhale hiss move to a tall kneeing position.

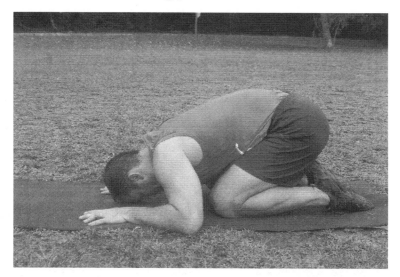

- From the tall kneeling position contract the glutes. Breathe in bracing the abdominals, lean back rounding the spine and neck looking up. Place your hands on your lower back for support if needed. Perform for 3-5 breathing cycles and on the exhale hiss move back to the center. You want to breathe in to keep the abdominals and pressure active to support and stabilize the lower back.

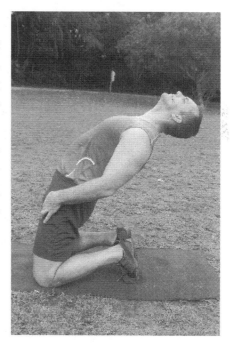

Without breathing in, you lose pressure that produces excessive force, compressing the vertebra of the lumbar lower back. Contracting the gluts produces the platform of stability for the lumbar and prevents excessive force to the lumbar. Remember this rule when perform hyperextension movements.

Kneeling Arm Bar Rotation

- From the kneeling position, put one hand on the floor in front of you and the other arm behind your back You can put you palm against the body or open turned out.
- Breathe in and push the hand into the floor isometrically, rotating the head and spine to the arm bar side contracting the neck, shoulder, lat and the opposing oblique muscles. Focus on moving the elbow in the rotation toward the spine. Focus on the X Movement Pattern (right oblique, left shoulder and vise versa). Perform 3-5 breathing cycles with the rotation.
- Exhale hiss and move back to center. Perform the other side.
- Repeat 3-5 times on each side.

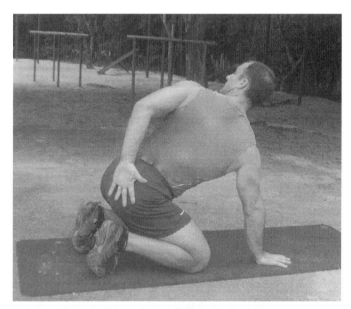

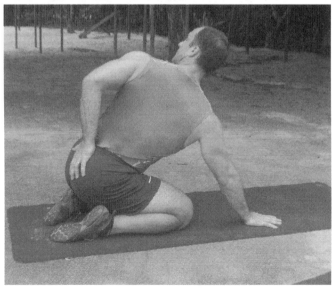

High Kneeling Spinal Rotation

- Choose your position with knees together (top photos) or the bottom photos with knees apart.
- Place your arms in front of you. Contract the glutes, breathe in and rotate the spine to one side. Using the X movement pattern, contract the oblique and the opposite side lat. Do not try to rotate too much. Just let your brain feel the muscles contract to guide the motion. Once they can guide the motion, you will improve range of motion. Perform 3-5 breathing cycles in the rotation with the contraction of the lat and oblique. On the final exhale hiss, move back to the center position and perform the other side.
- Alternate side to side 3-5 times.

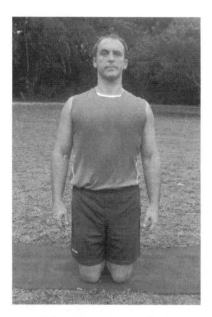 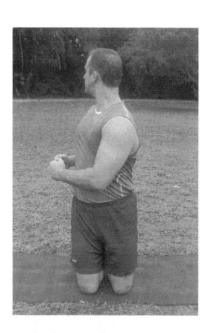

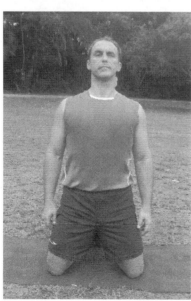 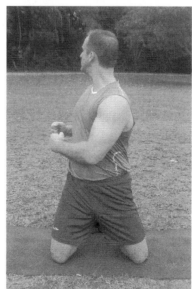

Cervical Lat Tension Flexion Hyperextension

Go slow and don't force these movements. Pull the shoulders down and pull the elbows into your ribcage to activate the lat's during the cervical movements.

- Breathe in and touch the chin to the top of the chest to contract the muscles in the front and stretch the back of the neck. Perform 3-5 breathing cycles. Exhale hiss and move the head back to center.

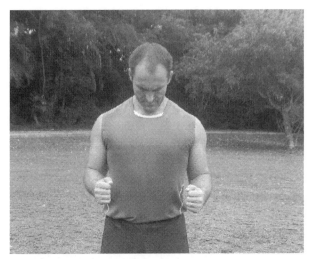

- Breathe in and look up contracting the back of the neck and stretching the front of the neck. Perform 3-5 breathing cycles. When looking down and up, keep your teeth together not apart for optimal stretch and contraction in the neck.

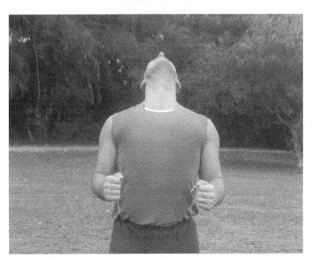

Don't compensate alignment by rounding your spine or rolling the shoulders forward to do the motions. If you cannot touch the chin to your chest, you need to contract and strengthen those neck muscles to do it. You should feel the muscles in the back of the neck stretching and vise versa. Keep good posture or you will not feel the motions. Go through the cervical movements slowly focusing on contracting one side and stretching the other.

Cervical Lat Tension Side Bend Rotations

- Pull the shoulders down, and elbows into the ribcage to contract the lat's.
- Breathe in and bend the neck laterally to one side. Hold the position and perform 3-5 breathing cycles along with contracting the lat's.
- Exhale hiss back to center. Then breathe in and rotate to the opposite side. Hold the position for 3-5 breathing cycles contracting the lat's. Perform other side.
- GO Slow! Don't force. Complete 3-5 times on each side alternating side to side to feel for asymmetry and work longer on it. Function first.

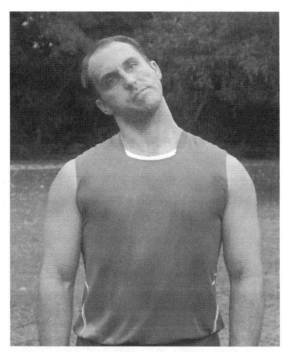

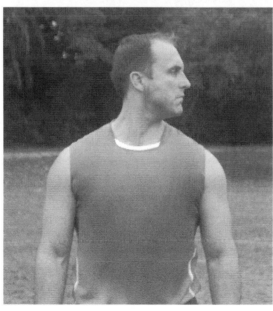

Cervical Chin Touch (11-5) (1-7)

- Turn your head into an 11 o'clock position and touch your chin to your collarbone. Try to touch without compensating rounding the spine to do it. Perform 3-5 breathing cycles. On the inhalation, look up tilt the head back into to the 5 O'clock position and perform 3-5 breathing cycles. Exhale hiss and return to the center position.

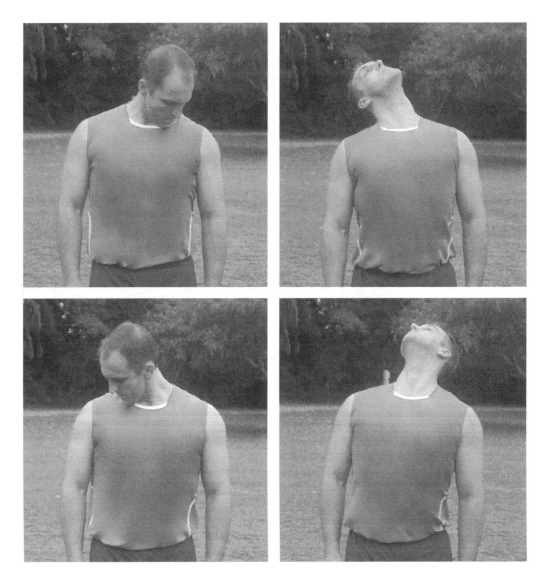

- Rotate your head into a 1 O'clock position and touch your chin to your collarbone. Try to touch without compensating rounding the spine to do it. Perform 3-5 breathing cycles. On the inhalation, look up tilt the head back into to the 7 O'clock position and perform 3-5 breathing cycles. Exhale hiss and return to the center position. Perform and alternate 3-5 times.

Cervical Shrug Up Retract Rotation

- Look up tilt the head back and shrug the shoulders up contracting the back of the neck muscles and traps. Perform 3-5 breathing cycles.

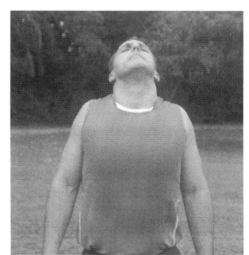

- Then retract the shoulders contracting the lats rotating the head to the left at the same time. Perform 3-5 breathing cycles holding the position

- Lift up contract look up. Perform 3-5 breathing cycles.

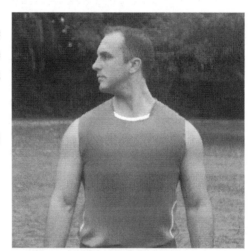

- Retract and rotate to the right. Perform 3-5 breathing cycles.

- Repeat 3-5 times the whole sequence.

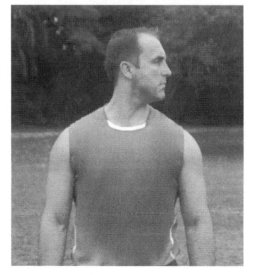

Kneeling on Hands Cervical Rotation

- From the kneeling position sitting on your heels, lean on your hands, putting pressure into the floor. This will activate the lats, triceps, shoulders and abdominals. Perform 3-5 breathing cycles.

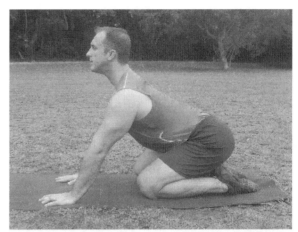

- Breathe in and rotate your head left. Hold the position and perform 3-5 breathing cycles. Exhale hiss back to center.

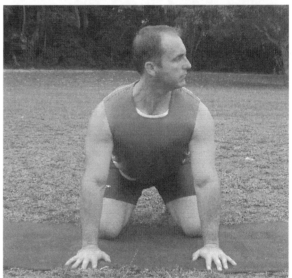

- Breathe in and rotate your head right. Perform 3-5 breathing cycles. Exhale hiss back to center.

- Repeat 3-5 times the whole sequence.

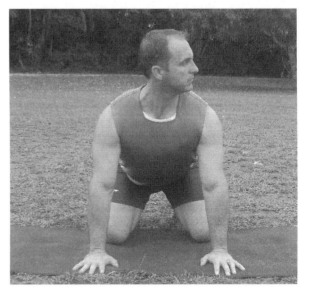

Lying Down Knee Rolls

- Lying on your back with your knees up and feet flat on the floor, breathe in and lift your knees up slowly rolling them toward the chest lifting the hip off the floor. Only roll the knees to the point to where your back stays flat on the floor.
- Perform 3-5 breathing cycles pulling the knees up to the chest. After 3-5 breathing cycles lower the feet to the floor.

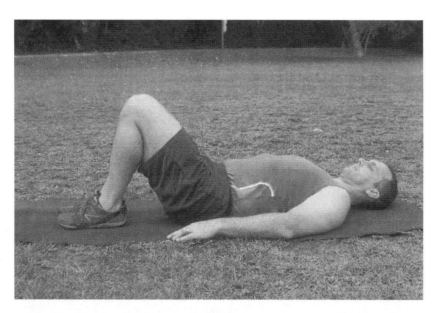

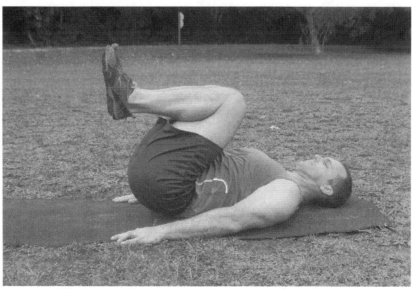

Straight Back Sit Up Knees Bent

- Lying on your back with your knees up and feet flat on the floor, breathe in and lift your torso off the floor. Don't worry about the height that you can lift. Focus on lifting with a straight aligned spine. Lift your chest up parallel to the ceiling, not rounding your spine forward.

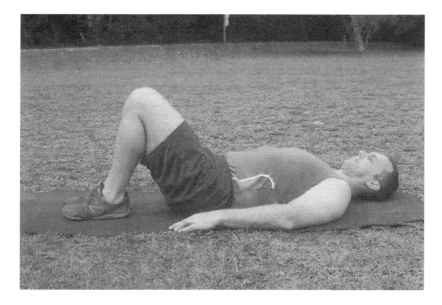

- Focus on lifting your chest and it will contract the spine muscles with the abdominals. Don't do crunches! Perform 3-5 breathing cycles holding the up lifted position. Then, exhale hiss and lower down to the floor.
- Repeat 3-5 times.

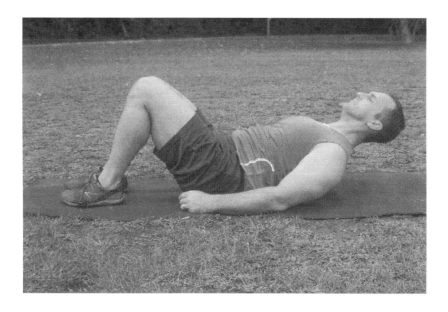

Lying Down Alternate Knee Lift Leg Extension Up

- Lying on your back with your knees up and feet flat on the floor, breathe in and lift your knees up slowly rolling them toward the chest lifting the hips off the floor (side photo). Only roll the knees to the point to where your back stays flat on the floor. Perform 3-5 breathing cycles.

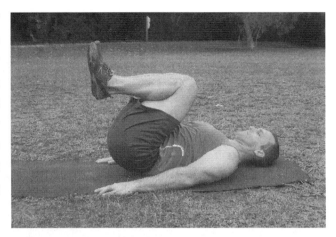

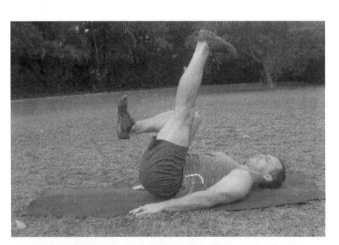

- Extend one leg contracting the quads, abs and slightly pulling the toes toward the knee. As one leg is extended up, keep the bent knee active pulling toward the chest. Perform 3-5 breathing cycles with the leg in the extended position and switch legs to do the same. Alternate side-to-side performing 3-5 breathing cycles as one rep.

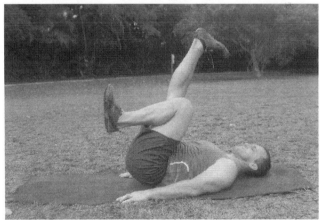

- Perform 3-5 times on each leg.

Straight Back Sit Up Alternate Single Leg Lever

- Laying on your back breathe in and lift up into a straight back sit up position with both knees bent and feet on the floor. Secure this position. Perform 3-5 breathing cycles.

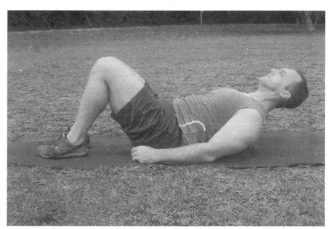

- Holding the straight back up off the floor, straighten one leg into a lever position contracting the quads, glutes and abs, slightly pulling the toes toward the knee. Perform 3-5 breathing cycles. Place the foot on the floor and extend the other.

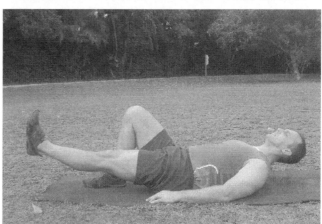

- Straighten the other leg into a lever position contracting the quads, glutes and abs, slightly pulling the toes toward the knee. Perform 3-5 breathing cycles. Place the foot on the floor.

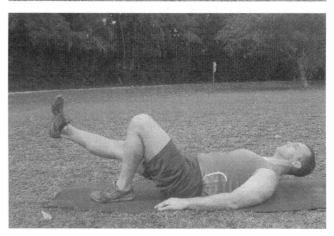

- Repeat alternating 3-5 times.

Straight Back Sit Up Single Leg Lever Leg Extension Up

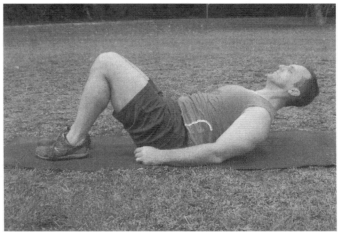

- Lying on your back breathe in and lift up into a straight back sit up position and hold that position.

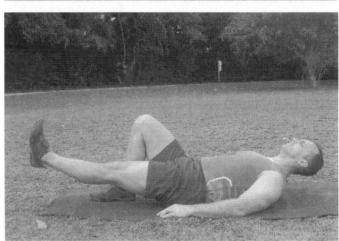

- Lever one leg straight contracting the quads, glutes and abs, slightly pulling the toes toward the knee. Perform 3-5 breathing cycles. Exhale hiss, lift and extend the leg up.

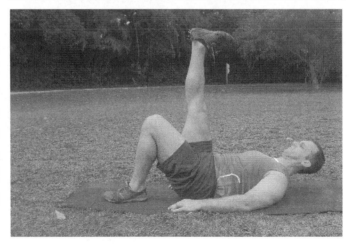

- Once the leg is extended up, maintain the quad contraction and the toes being pulled toward the knee to stretch the hamstring. Hold the extended leg position and perform 3-5 breathing cycles.

Straight Back Sit Up Double Leg Levers Leg Extensions Up

- Lying on your back breathe in and lift up into a straight back sit up position. Hold the position for 3-5 breathing cycles.

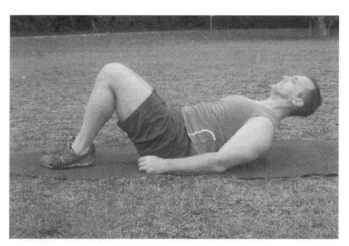

- Exhale hiss and extend both legs into a lever position contracting the glutes, quads and abs as you straighten the legs. Slightly pull the toes toward the knees. Perform 3-5 breathing cycles holding this position.

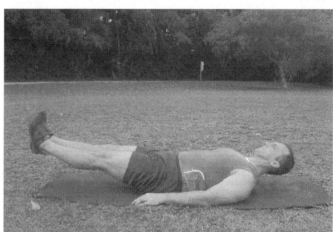

- From the leg lever position Exhale hiss and lift the legs straight up, contracting the quads, abs and slightly pulling the toes toward the knees. Perform for 3-5 breathing cycles. Repeat 3-5 times each position with the breathing cycles.

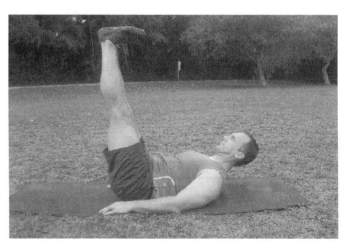

Side Plank

- Get into a side position using your hand or your elbow, positioning it under your shoulder. Stack your feet on top of each other.
- Breathe in and lift the hips up. Brace the abdominals with your hips in the midline position. Perform 3-5 breathing cycles holding this position. After 3-5 breathing cycles, exhale hiss and lower your self down to the floor and perform the other side.
- Repeat alternating side to side 3-5 times.

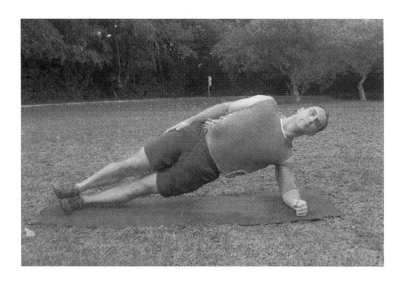

Side Plank (Foot Assist)

- If you are having problems stacking your feet or to maintain balance and stability, use this side plank formation. Bring the top leg forward and place the foot flat on the floor. Push through the foot pushing your hip up to the ceiling and follow the same breathing technique. Perform the same as above.

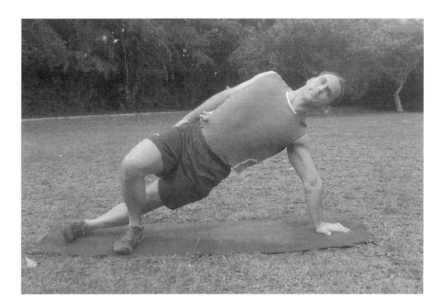

Side Plank Leg Lift

- Get into a side position using a hand or elbow position under your shoulder. Stack your feet on top of each other. Breathe in and lift your hips up contracting the oblique, lat and shoulder on the planked arm. Perform 3-5 breathing cycles in the neutral position.

- Once you have established position, exhale hiss and lift the leg up and perform 3-5 breathing cycles with the leg up. On the exhale hiss lower the leg down and perform the other side. Repeat alternating side to side 3-5 times and holding longer any weakness.

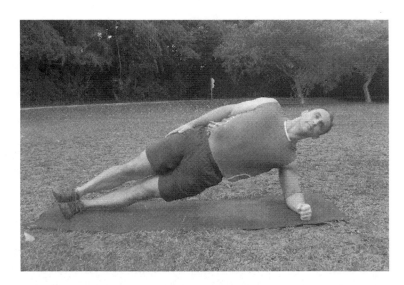

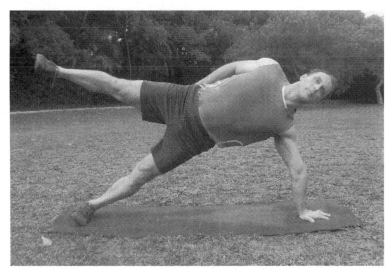

Side Plank Leg Lift Arm Reach

- Get into a side position using a hand or elbow position under your shoulder. Stack your feet on top of each other. Breathe in lifting the hips up into the air contracting the oblique, lat and shoulder on the planked arm. Perform 3-5 breathing cycles in the neutral position.

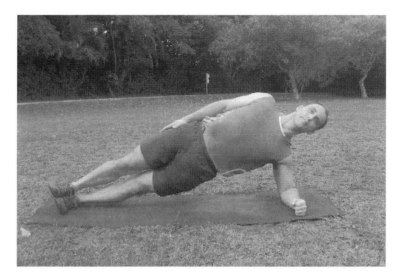

- Once you have established position exhale hiss and lift the leg up and reach the arm overhead. Stabilize the position and perform 3-5 breathing cycles contracting all the muscles at the same time. On the exhale hiss, lower the leg return the arm back to the side position and lower the hips down to the floor. Perform the other side.
- Repeat alternating side to side 3-5 times.

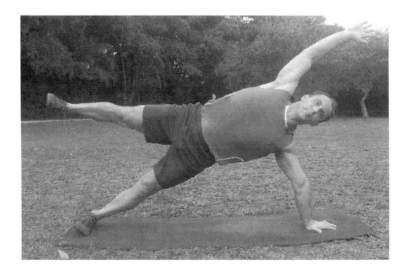

Side Plank Leg Lift Arm Reach Elbow Knee Touch

Now that you have balance and stability, you can now coordinate movement.

- Get into a side plank position. Stack your feet on top of each other. Breathe in lifting the hips up into the air contracting the muscles on the planked arm. Perform 3-5 breathing cycles.

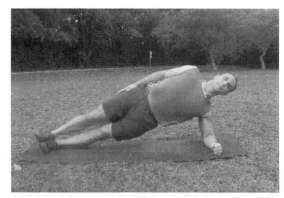

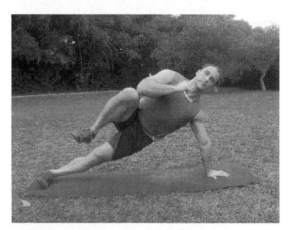

- Breathe in and touch the elbow and knee together. You can use the same side or opposites to touch.

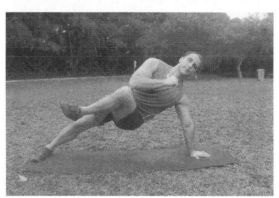

185

- After touching the elbow and knee, exhale hiss extend the leg and reach the arm overhead. Hold for 3-5 breathing cycles. Breathe in brace and lower the leg and bring the arm back to the side. Exhale hiss and lower the hips down to the floor. Perform the other side.
- Repeat alternating side to side for **3-5 repetitions**.

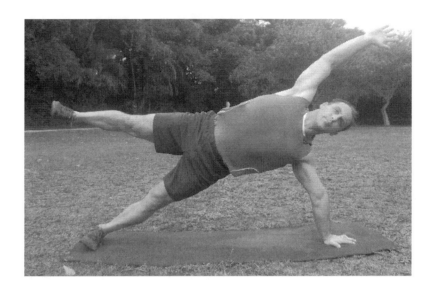

Always focus on control to improve proprioception for strong movement.

Side Plank Elbow Knee Touch Leg Extension

- Get into a side position using a hand or elbow position under your shoulder. Stack your feet on top of each other. Breathe in lifting the hips up into the air contracting the muscles on the planked arm. Perform 3-5 breathing cycles.

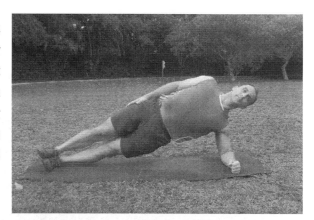

- Breathe in touching the knee and elbow.

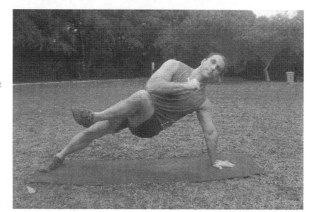

- Then, exhale hiss reaching the arm overhead and extend the leg in front of you contracting the quads and slightly pulling the toes toward the knee. Hold and perform 3-5 breathing cycles.

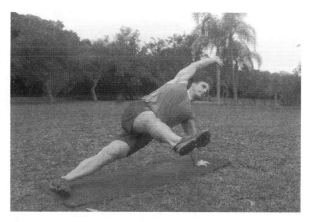

- Exhale hiss and return the arm to the side and bring the leg back down to the floor as in photo one. Perform the other side. **Repeat 3-5 times alternating side to side.**

Bird Dog

- If you cannot do the plank, position yourself on all fours, on your hands and knees, maintaining a straight spine.
- Breathe in and push your hands into the floor to contract the lat's and triceps. Exhale hiss and extend the arm straight above your head, contracting the lat, shoulder and triceps and the lift the opposing leg, contracting the quads and glutes, keeping the foot straight. Perform for 3-5 breathing cycles and then bring the hand and knee back to position. Perform the other side.
- Alternate side to side for 3 -5 repetitions.

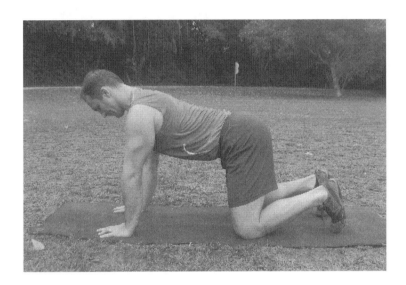

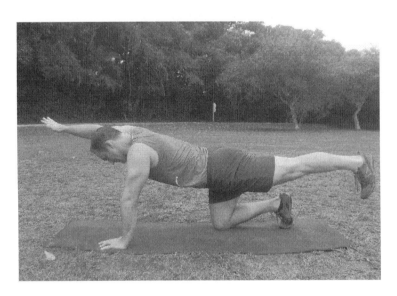

Plank

- Laying face down on the floor, breathe in and lift yourself up into a plank position.
- Contract the glutes, quads lats and triceps. Hold and perform 3 to 5 breathing cycles then exhale hiss and relax the muscles.

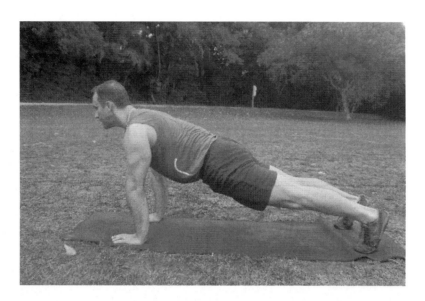

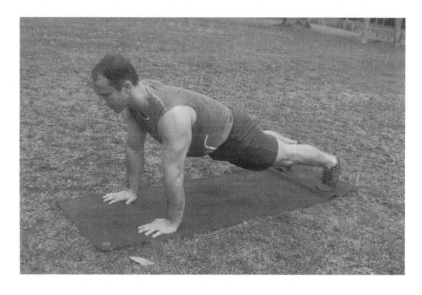

Alternating One Arm Plank Walk Up Overhead

- Laying face down on the floor, breathe in and lift yourself up into a plank position. Contract the glutes, quads, lats and triceps.
- Exhale hiss and walk one arm /hand up. Maintain the glute and quad contraction and perform 3-5 breathing cycles. You can use both hands as well.
- Breathe in back to the start position and move the other hand up. Perform 3-5 breathing cycles. Repeat 3-5 times on each arm.

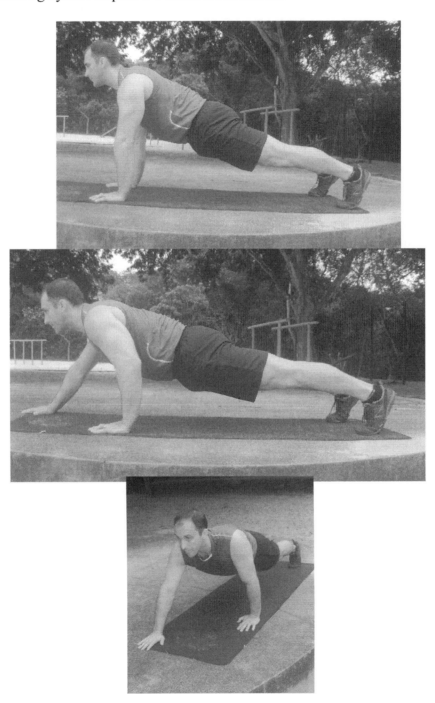

Plank Leg Lifts

- From the plank position, breathe in contract and compress. Perform 3-5 breathing cycles.
- Exhale hiss lifting one leg up and perform 3-5 breathing cycles.

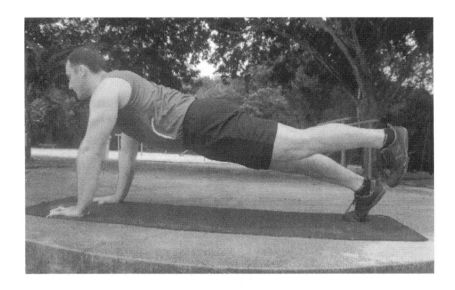

- Then move the leg away from the body. Contract the glutes and quads on the straight leg on the floor to stabilize the power and coordination of lifting the leg up and away. Feel the glute medius on the side of the hip contract as you move the leg away from the body. Keep the quads tight as well. Perform 3-5 breathing cycles holding the leg out to the side contracting the quads and glutes. Maintain spine and hip alignment.

- Repeat the sequence 3-5 times.

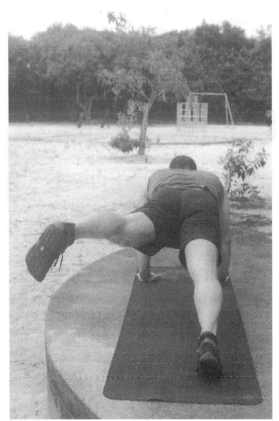

Plank Opposite Arm and Leg Lift

- From the plank position, contract and compress for 3-5 breathing cycles.
- Exhale hiss lifting one leg and the opposite arm off up off the floor. Contract the glutes and quads on the straight leg on the floor to stabilize the power and coordination of lifting the leg, and contract the quads and glutes on the lifted leg as well.
- Contract the lats and triceps on both arms the stabilizing arm and the lifted arm. Perform 3-5 breathing cycles holding the position.
- Exhale hiss and lower the arm and leg back to the position. Perform the other side. Alternate side-to-side performing slowly or you can work one side only first. Use your breathing to increase the power of stability and to relax at the same time.
- Repeat 3-5 times each side.

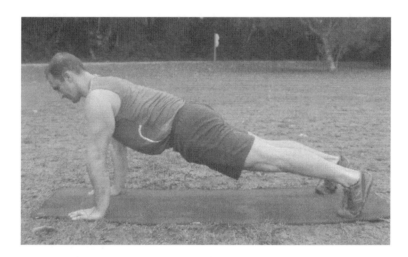

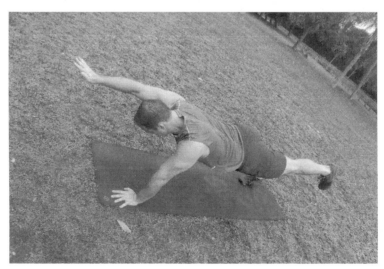

Reverse Plank and Reverse Plank Scissors

- Sitting on the floor with the fingers turned away from the body and legs in front, breathe in and then exhale hiss and lift your body up into the air toward the ceiling into a reverse plank position.

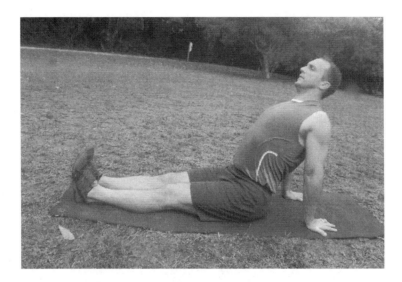

- Contract the quads and glutes to help keep the hips up. Lift your chest up to the ceiling and let the shoulder blades try to touch. This will help keep the lats, shoulders and triceps contracted. Perform 3-5 breathing cycles in this contracted position. On the exhale hiss relax and lower the body down to the floor.
- Repeat 3-5 times.

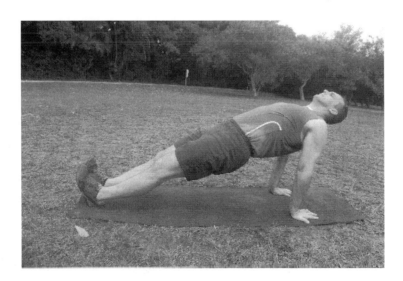

- You can perform the same pose using a scissor position with the legs. You can also add a challenge by lifting one leg up and out to the side, alternating side-to-side.

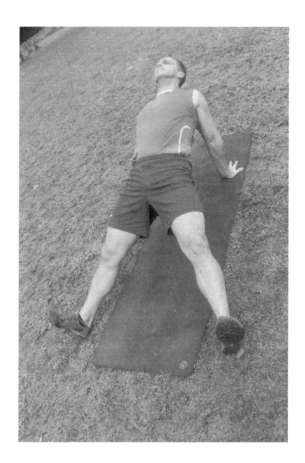

Arm Bar Waist Wrap Cervical Rotation

- From a standing position, breathe in, lift your chest, slide you hand and arm behind your lower back to the other side of your hip and rotate your head to the side your arm is behind the back. Contract the lat, shoulder and neck muscles.
- Once you have position, perform 3-5 breathing cycles rotating the head, contracting the muscles and then switch sides.

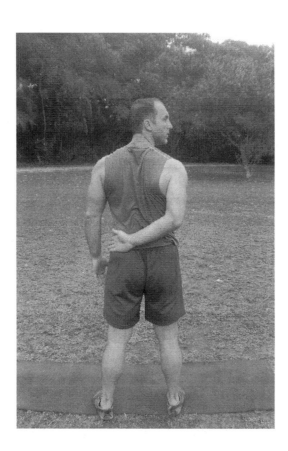

Arm Bar Mid Back Lift Arm Extension Cervical Rotation

- Breathe in and place your arm behind your back with the palm facing away from the body. Try not to rest the arm on the back because you will relax the muscles needed to develop strength in the movement.
- Rotate the head contracting the neck muscles to the same side the arm is reaching. Perform 3-5 breathing cycles with the arm behind the back.
- Exhale hiss and extend your arm contracting your triceps with the palm up. Perform 3-5 breathing cycles with the arm in the extended position reaching back. Breathe in and return the arm to the mid-back.
- Repeat each motion 3-5 times.

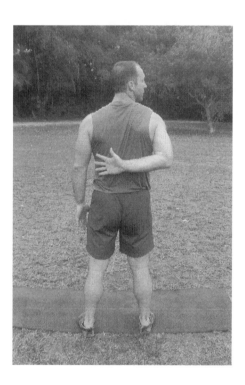 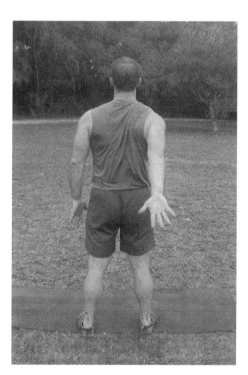

Remember a small amount of movement is a lot for strength and alignment development.

Arm Bar Lift Extension Side Rotation

- Breathe in and place your arm behind your back with the palm facing away from the body. Perform 3-5 breathing cycles.
- Exhale hiss and extend your arm behind you with the palm up contracting the triceps, lats and back of the shoulder. Perform 3-5 breathing cycles.

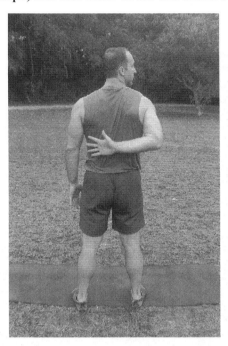 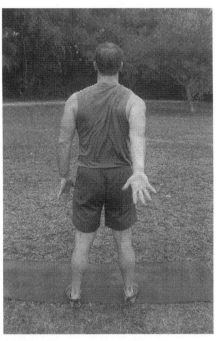

- Exhale hiss and move the arm to the side position palm up. Perform 3-5 breathing cycles. Breathe in and return the arm to the mid-back position.
- Repeat 3-5 times

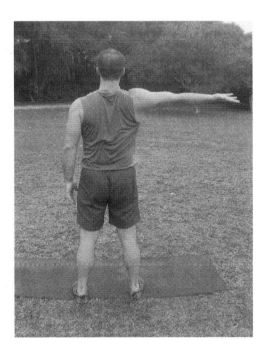

Arm Bar Extension Side Rotation Sword Drawl

- Breathe in and reach the backside of the palm across the back. Perform 3-5 breathing cycles.
- Exhale hiss and extend the arm straight contracting the triceps locking the elbow with the palm up. Perform 3-5 breathing cycles.

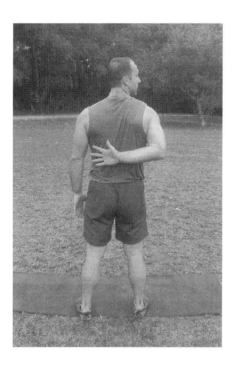 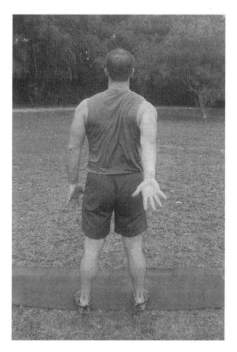

- Breathe in and turn the palm up lifting the arm straight out to the side with the palm facing up. Perform 3-5 breathing cycles.

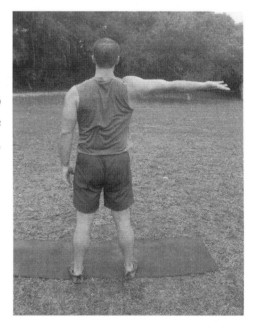

- Breathe in and reach your hand behind your neck maintaining neck and spine alignment. Perform 3-5 breathing cycles.

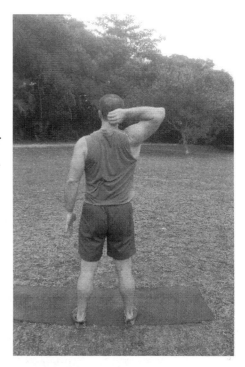

- Exhale hiss and reach into a Y position contracting the triceps and lats. Perform 3-5 breathing cycles.

- Repeat 3-5 times slowly contracting the muscles to guide the joints.

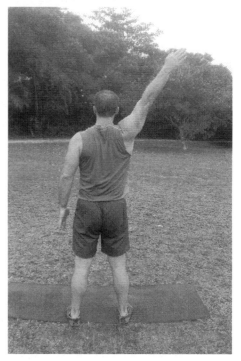

If you have to compensate your posture and shoulder joint to do move, then muscles are not contracting or there is misalignment. The only thing that should be moving is the arm and shoulder joint. Focus on contracting muscles and doing the movement slow.

Upright Row High Pull

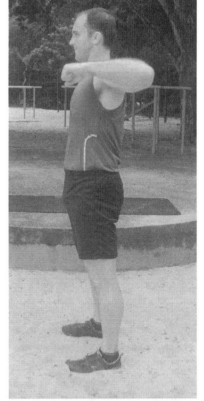

- Breathe in and pull your elbows back into a 90-degree position with the body. Contract the lats and the back of the shoulders. Keep the neck in an aligned position. Perform 3-5 breathing cycles with pulling the elbows back.

- Once you have a tight compressed position breathe in and roll the wrist down pulling back with the elbows. Perform 3-5 breathing cycles with the wrist down. Repeat for 3-5 reps each position.

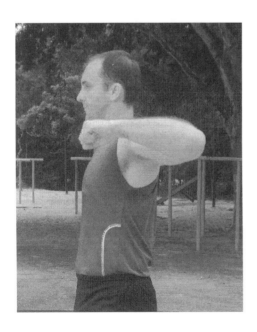

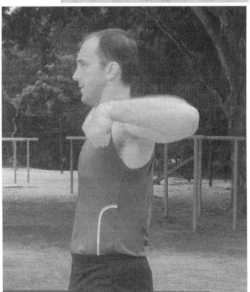

T's

- Place the arms out to the sides with palms facing forward. Keep the elbows locked to contract the triceps.
- Breathe in and slowly pull the arms back at the same time pulling back the fingers. Pulling back the fingers is the key to this exercise. Feel the forearm muscles contract.
- Perform 3-5 breathing cycles once you have position. Exhale hiss and relax. Repeat 3-5 times.

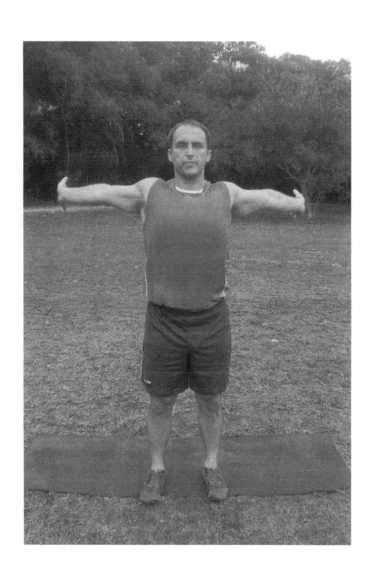

Karate Punches

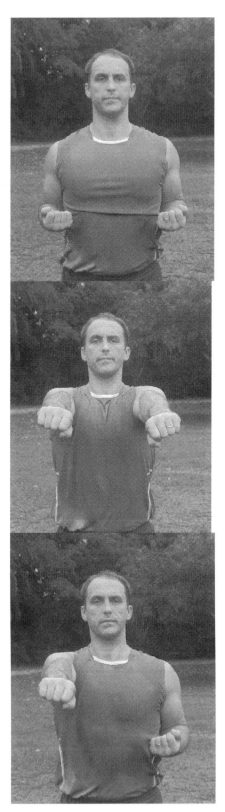

- Make a fist and position your arms at a 90-degree angle with the palms facing up, pulling the elbow into the rib cage to engage the lats, shoulders and back muscles. Perform 3 to 5 breathing cycles.

- Exhale hiss rotating both palms downward and extend the arms straight out in front of you. Contract the chest, back, triceps and shoulders from up to down in an extended position. Perform 3-5 breathing cycles. Don't just move contract the muscles.

- You can also do one arm at a time. As you extend one arm, pull the bent arm into the ribcage to contract the lats. Perform 3-5 breathing cycles and then switch arms.

- Repeat 3-5 times each side.

Chicken Wings Up and Down

- Standing up or sitting down keep good posture. Breathe in and clasp your fingers behind your head, pull your elbows back and squeeze the trapezius muscles below the neck, the back of the shoulders and lats. Perform 3-5 breathing cycles as you try to touch the elbows. Make sure you connect the contraction and stretch with the breathing and abdominal brace. If you are standing up contract the glutes. After 3-5 breathing cycles exhale hiss and relax.

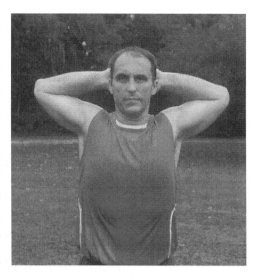

- Now place your hands on your lower back with fingers pointed down. Breathe in and pull the elbows back. Feel the lats and shoulders contract with the breath, tightening the abdominals. Perform 3-5 breathing cycles. Don't hyperextend the spine. (This will compensate the shoulders alignment. If you hyperextend the spine you will not feel the exercise as much and have false mobility.) Pull the elbows toward each other.

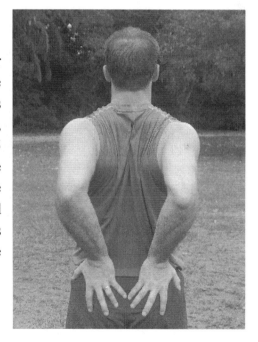

- Repeat alternating up and down 3-5 times.

Wrist Figure 8's

- Clasp you hands and fingers together. Start rolling the wrist slowly in a figure 8 motion. Try not to let the palms separate. One wrist bends and rolls up the other down.
- Keep rolling them alternating them up and down. Start slow and find the barriers of tension producing poor mobility.
- Perform 5 reps or more one way then perform the other way.

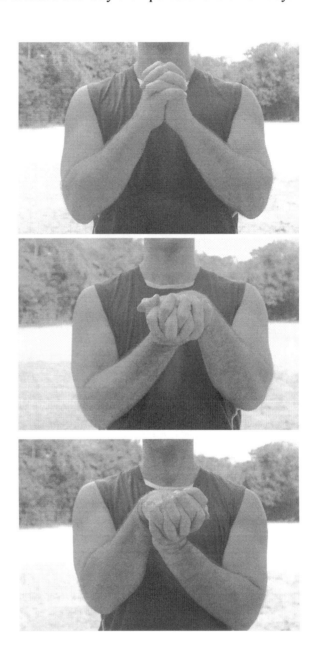

Floor Desk Stretch

- On your hands and knees place the hands flat on the floor. Or from the standing position place your hands on a desk or table with the palms facing away. Contract the triceps and contract the opposite side of the forearm muscles to facilitate stretch opening the space of the joint. Perform 3-5 breathing cycles.

- Stretch by leaning the body back toward the feet into the fingers pointing toward the body. Do it slowly and try to keep the palms flat. Hold and perform 3-5 breathing cycles. Don't force. More space will open or it will feel more comfortable.

- Repeat 3-5 times.

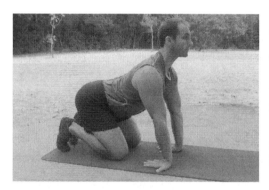 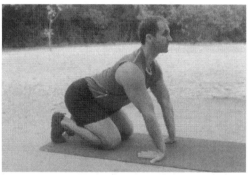

- Switch the hand position turning the fingers away from you and perform the same process as above. Except now move your body over your wrist.

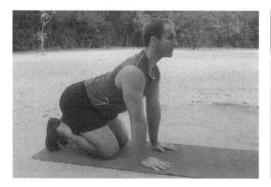 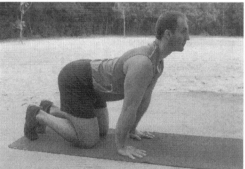

Straight Arm Wrist Fist Flexion Rotation

- With your arms at your side make a fist and curl the wrist back, palm up. If you slouch the shoulders you will not feel the movement as much. Make a tight fist and contract the triceps and forearm muscles. Feel the stretch in the front of the wrist from just contracting the triceps. Now rotate the shoulder and wrist back to front with emphasis on pointing the wrist toward the floor. Rotate the hand forward so the palm is still up. When you rotate, the fist will pass close to the body.
- Repeat 3- 5 times.

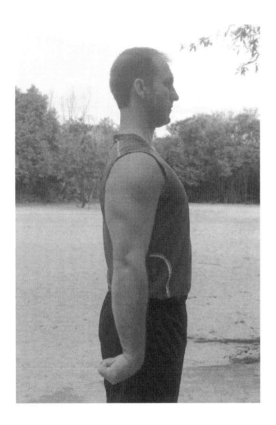 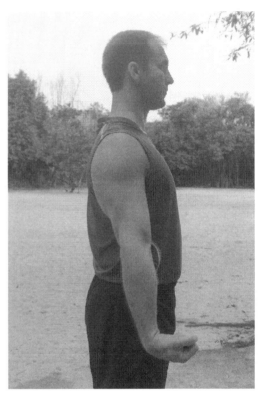

Fist to Finger Flexion Extensions

- Make a tight fist for 3-5 breathing cycles. Then extend the fingers wide, extending all the fingers away from each other. You should feel the fingers stretching and the webbing in between the fingers stretching as well.
- Hold the stretch for 3-5 breathing cycles.
- Repeat 3-5 times.

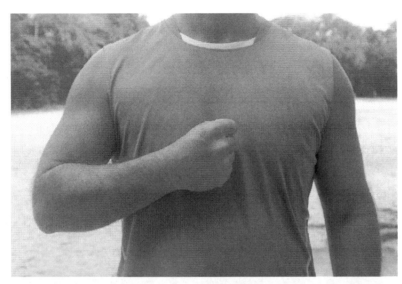

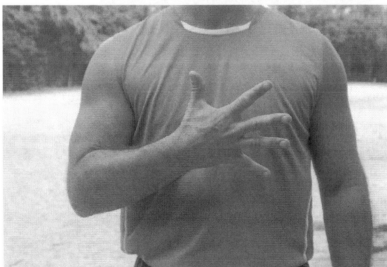

Finger Curls with Fingers Extended

- Stretch and extend the fingers away from each other. Starting with the index finger through to the pinky. When you curl one finger down, keep extending the fingers trying not to let them move. Perform 3-5 breathing cycles with each finger and hold the contracted finger.
- You can perform circles with each finger as well, while keeping the rest of the fingers extended.

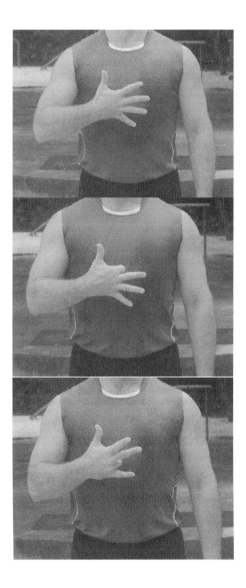 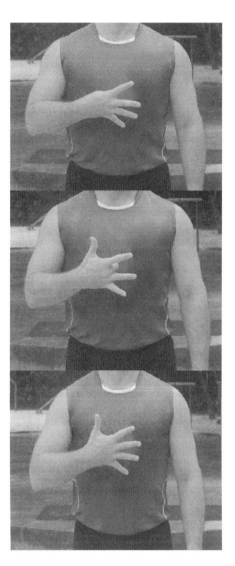

Plank Compression Pushup

- Breathe in and lower yourself down to the floor from the plank position. Keep the glute contracted

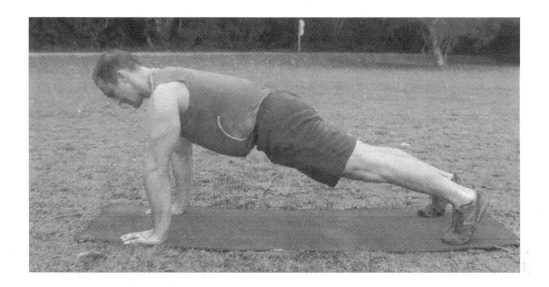

- Exhale hiss and push up from the floor. Keep the muscles compressed for tension.

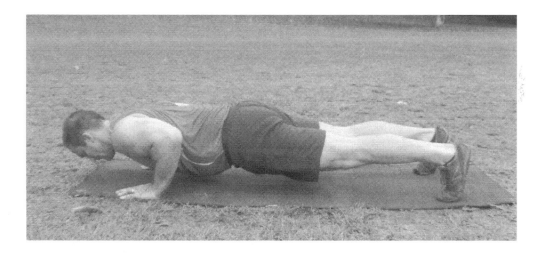

Eccentric Pushup or (From Knees)

- Hold the plank and perform 3-5 breathing cycles compressing and contracting the muscles.
- Breathe in and slowly lower yourself to the floor keeping everything contracted and tight without pushing up.

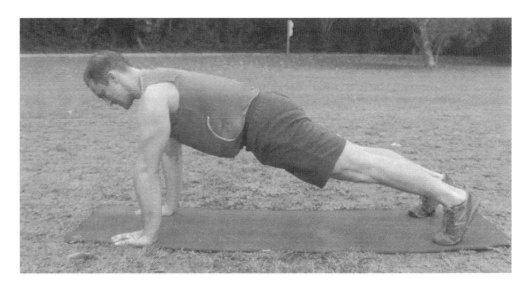

- Exhale hiss and lay on the floor.

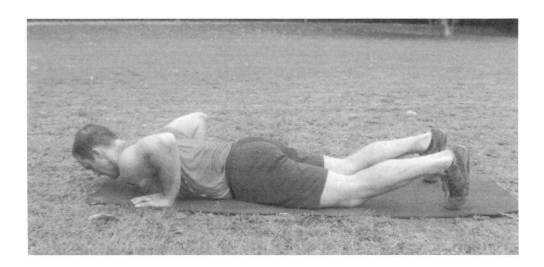

- Reset the plank position. Perform the movement slow contracting and compressing and you will be doing a pushup in no time quickly. Repeat 3-5 times.

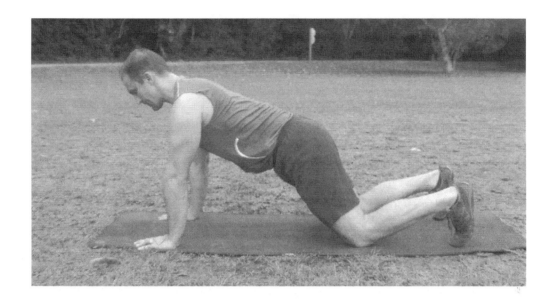

Star Plank Pushup

- Spread the legs open contracting the glut medius, buttock and the quadriceps. Hold the position for 3-5 breathing cycles and then perform a pushup.
- Breathe in lowering yourself down to the floor.
- As you get down to the floor hold the plank position and perform 3-5 breathing cycles. Exhale hiss and pushup up. As you exhale and push up, contract the muscles tight.
- Perform 3-5 repetitions.

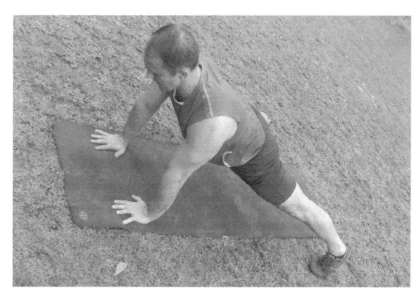

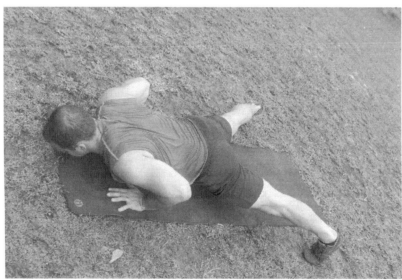

Triangle Pushup

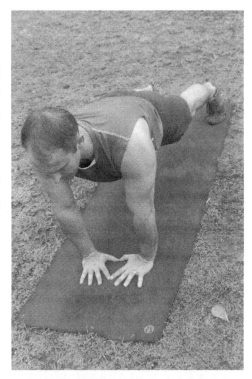

- Create a triangle with your thumb and index finger to perform a pushup. The triangle should be lined up with the sternum, the middle of the chest.

- Contract the quads and glutes and hold the triangle plank position for 3-5 breathing cycles.

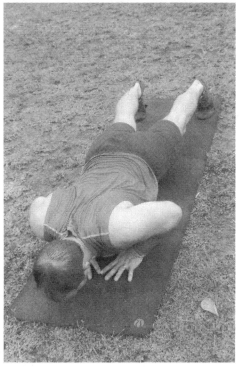

- Breathe in and lower yourself down to the floor keeping all the muscles contracted.

- At the bottom hold for 3-5 breathing cycles and then on the exhale hiss pushup up. Perform slow repetitions contracting the quads, glutes, lats and triceps.

- Repeat 3-5 times.

CONCLUSION

"Stepping onto a brand-new path is difficult, but not more difficult than remaining in a situation, that is not nurturing to the whole woman." – Maya Angleou

In a world plagued by pain, injury, disorder and disease, we need prevention. In order to obtain health, fitness, youth and vitality in our life we need to use our essential and powerful resources of breathing and alignment. Like screening for cardiovascular disease before exercise, we need to screen how we are breathing and the position of our joints. By screening and understanding our breathing and alignment for health or before exercise, fitness or performance, we can discover the detrimental, malfunctioning, harmful and unhealthy issues that produce strain, pain and injury and prevent them. When we function optimally, have energy and health, we open life's opportunities by maintaining our youthful interests slowing down the aging process. By making this information more mainstream to doctors, surgeons, physical therapist, trainers, anyone in bodywork, the medical profession, athletes or just out to the general public, we can begin to change statistics to pain, injury and disorders, especially musculoskeletal ones. We can produce a healthier society. But it all starts with you making a difference. Be mindful to make changes in your lifestyle and better choices to how you live. Becoming conscious and aware to our unconscious habits and programing develops our life to be more effective, and goes beyond just discovering health. Being mindful helps us adapt, adjust and change, to evolve a new self.

Be mindful about how you are functioning, about the condition of your energy, how you are feeling each day and focus on changing the issues that are disrupting your happiness, energy, enjoyment and wellness to live at this very moment. If you are not functional, you fall behind on the path of progression and evolution. Falling behind leads you to seek out ways and methods to catch up using devices, pills, drinks, medications and misinformation that is more attractive than beneficial. Take time to understand yourself and your weaknesses because the weaknesses make your strengths and life less efficient and less effective anchoring your potential. Lack of mindfulness allows poor quality to exist, leaving you stuck in the past, losing the ability to adapt, adjust and change. Everyone should have the potential to learn how to fix him or herself and move well. One must have time to learn, to understand the idea of change through time. J. Krishnamurti said, in *This Light in Oneself*, "When we take time to learn, we put all the systems and functions into perspective that integrate to build each other to accomplish a goal or intention." There are things functioning and happening beyond our awareness. Our job is to understand these things and bring them into our consciousness, educate them and train them. Being aware, mindful and conscious affects the present to change the future of our health and longevity as a society or an individual. We can't just assume we were born to move well. We can't just assume we are healthy. Life happened and limitations took hold, producing a lost path that could not return to its natural course. What is present today creates the advantages or disadvantages for tomorrow, producing a healthy or diseased and disordered longevity.

We are always seeking how to be better but often forget the simple, natural and effortless path to take us there. We miss the point about our functional qualities and the foundational building blocks that form health and movement. We forget that many things integrate in life, to create and give power to the whole. We subject ourselves to the most powerful things without having the proper thoughts, intentions and circuitry to plug us in. Most people can't simply master breathing functionally to make it healthy and well. Most people can't maintain alignment to avoid pain and strain but yet they want to be healthy and strong. It is not the greatest thing on the market that everyone needs to be strong and healthy. You must prepare yourself to move forward so that the functions fit the movement process, the training, so it becomes natural and effortless each day and not a struggle to practice. Change your thinking to take charge of your health. Be mindful. Breathe more. Exercise more. Meditate. Sleep and eat well. These qualities are how we connect to our health, youth, vitality and energy for longevity to evolve the mind, body and spirit (MBS) for life.

MBS is a cycle of integration that affects each other. If you are happy, sad, healthy, youthful, in pain, it goes through the cycle affecting the mind, body and spirit, like a spinning wheel. Is the wheel bent and wobbly or trued and centered? Choose things that are positive to go into the cycle to keep the MBS operating and integrating (spinning) smoothly to preserve the true center and function. The bent wheel needs to be fixed in order to perform or improve performance or else you ride through life uncomfortably and at risk. It's not just about living longer it's about living better, extracting the things that interrupt the cycle's performance, producing poor qualities, compensated and dysfunctional. This is the purpose of *The Balanced Body*: simple preventative medicine for life. Master simplicity, for it holds all the answers to life, fitness, performance, health, youth, vitality and happiness.

"The world as we have created it is a process of our thinking. It cannot be changed without changing our thinking." – Albert Einstein

References

Marcus, Dr. Norman. *End Back Pain Forever: A Ground Breaking Approach to Eliminate Your Suffering*. New York: Atria Books, 2012.

McGill, Dr. Stuart. *Ultimate Back Fitness and Performance*. Champaign, IL: Stuart McGill Publishing, 2004.

Cook, Gray. FMS Certification: Stability /Mobility Chart

Simons M.D., David G., Travell M.D., Janet G., Simons P.T, Lois S. *Myofascial Pain and Dysfunction: The Trigger Point Manual, Volume One Upper Half of the Body*. Baltimore, MD: Williams and Wilkins, 1999.

Simons M.D., David G., Travell M.D., Janet G., Simons P.T, Lois S. *Myofascial Pain and Dysfunction: The Trigger Point Manual, Volume Two Lower Half of the Body*. Baltimore, MD: Williams and Wilkins, 1999.

Mark Kasmer, et. al., "Foot Strike Pattern and Gait Changes During a 161-km Ultramarathon," Journal of Strength and Conditioning Research, 28(5), 2014

Mangla PK, Menon MP. (1981, September 11). *Effect of Nasal and Oral Breathing on Exercise-Induced Asthma*. Retrieved from Pubmed.gov.

Dr. Mercola. (2013, November 24). *How the Buteyko Breathing Method Can Improve Your Health and Fitness*. Retrieved from Mercola.com

Jon Lundberg. (2008, November). *Nitric Oxide and the Paranasal sinuses*. Retrieved from Pubmed.gov.

Nattie E. (1999, November). CO_2, Brainstem Chemoreceptors and Breathing. Retrieved from Pubmed.gov.

Clifford PS, Hellsten Y. *"Vasodilatory Mechanisms in Contracting Skeletal Muscle,"* Journal of Applied Physiology, (1985).2004 Jul; 97(1):393-403.

James Knierim, Ph.D., Neuroscience Online Textbook, University of Texas UT Health, Chapter 5, Section 5.6, Cerebellum and Control Systems. Retrieved from neuroscience.uth.tmc.edu.com.

Exercise Index

About the Author

Jason Kelly graduated from Temple University in Exercise Science. He has been an exercise physiologist and massage therapist for over 19 years. He has worked with diabetes and cardiovascular disease programing; the geriatric, general and athletic populations designing prevention and strength programs; corporations teaching their employees how to stay healthy, move and exercise well and use better ergonomics in the workplace. As a fitness director he taught, strength, power and health comes from within, how you function and how you move, not just move. With this philosophy, he overhauled the entire program in the fitness facility with his functional mindset and approach that had instant success and results. He has taught numerous workshops to physical therapist, athletic trainers, massage therapist and to the general population. From working with a diversity of populations, he saw that prevention is rarely taught and misconception are widely accepted and used leading to high statistics of pain, injury, disease and disorder. Incorporating his years of skill and experience, he developed the *Breathe, Stabilize, Move Function First Method* to combat and resolve pain, injury, disease and disorders like musculoskeletal ones, for people to move well, freely and frequently. When you are functional, have alignment and breathe well, you move well developing prevention, health, fitness or strength in your life or sport. It does not matter who you are, young, old, athlete or not, you need to be functional first to have the shield of prevention and the balanced foundation to nurture movement and foster strength to cultivate their growth.

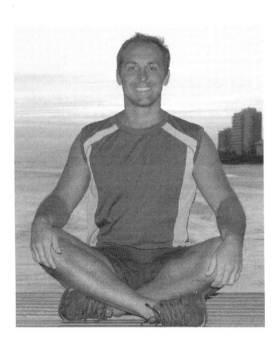

Made in the USA
Lexington, KY
04 May 2016